SEX

PLAY

SEX

PLAY

EMILY DUBBERLEY

De Vecchi
DVE Ediciones

BOOKINABOX

The right of Emily Dubberley to be identified as the author of the work has been asserted
by her in accordance with the Copyright, Designs and Patents Act 1988.

The author or publisher cannot be held responsible for the information (formulas, recipes, techniques, etc.) contained in the text, even though the utmost care has been taken in the writing of this work. In the case of specific - often unique - problems of each particular reader, it is advisable to consult a qualified person to obtain the most complete, accurate and up-to-date information possible. EDITORIAL DE VECCHI, S. A. U.

© Editorial De Vecchi, S. A. 2022
© [2022] Confidential Concepts International Ltd., Ireland
Subsidiary company of Confidential Concepts Inc, USA
ISBN: 978-1-63919-326-4

Contents

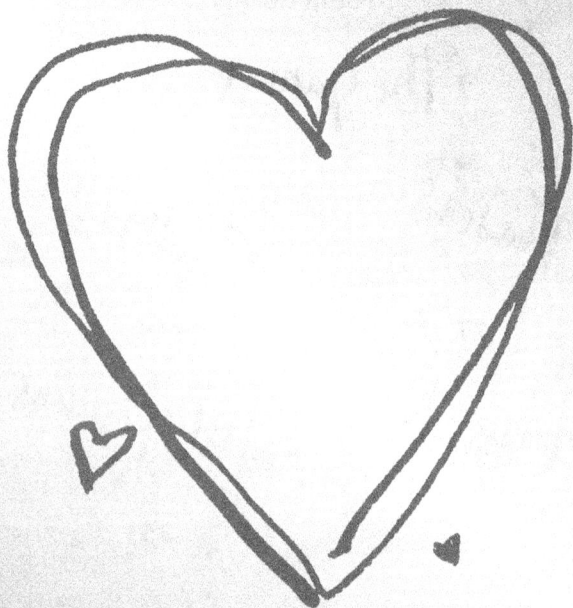

Introduction

It can be all too easy to slip into a routine in a relationship. Couples who play together stay together, and incorporating sexy games into your love life will help you keep things fresh. Just remember, it's about playing with each other – what could be sexier than that? By using dice – and plenty of imagination – Sex Play makes sex more of a game and, in doing so, helps you become the ultimate lover.

When was the last time you played a game? Maybe 'tag' at school? Or Trivial Pursuit after a dinner party? How about with your partner? In the bedroom? The chances are, you tend to focus on 'more important things' – like getting down and dirty. But playing games can help you to get even 'downer' and 'dirtier' – and, more to the point, help you to hone your sexual skills until your partner is quivering in anticipation at the mere thought of spending some quality time with you. All the games in *Sex Play* have been designed not only to work as foreplay, but also to help you learn about your partner and build on your sexual talents.

THE GAMES

Sex Play is divided into four groups of games: Teasers, Pleasing Him, Pleasing Her and Hot Positions. The Teasers can all be played fully clothed, and concentrate on helping you bond with your partner and learn about their greatest desires. Games in the Pleasing Him section are focused on giving a man sexual pleasure – although, if you're in a good relationship, hopefully you'll get pleasure from both giving and receiving sexual attention. Games in the Pleasing Her section concentrate on female enjoyment. And Hot Positions is packed with games to help you build up your repertoire of moves.

WHEN TO PLAY AND WITH WHOM

Sex Play is designed to be played by couples. Whether it's your first date or your fiftieth anniversary, you can use it to spice things up.

If you're in the early stages of a relationship, you may want to stick to the Teasers; as they've been designed to be played with clothes on, you won't find yourself in any position more compromising than kissing (or, at least, not because the cards have told you to …).

Pleasing Him and Pleasing Her focus on foreplay, so are ideal for evenings in together when you want to add extra spice to your night.

And Hot Positions are best tried either after you've completed games from the other sections, or after you've spent time on foreplay; only a quarter of women climax through penetrative sex alone, but, if a partner spends more than 20 minutes on foreplay, the figure increases to 90 per cent.

Other than that, there are no rules on when to play: you can go for a quick roll when you have a spare hour together, make a specific date of it, or play when you get back after a night out. You could take the box on holiday with you or keep it by the side of the bed to use whenever the mood takes you. If it's his birthday, treat him by using only the games for him, and vice versa. *Sex Play* is about having fun and learning more about each other; any time you're alone together can be the right time for that.

HOW TO PLAY

Start by rolling all three dice. Whoever has the highest score takes four of the envelopes from the front of the box. The other person takes five. Now, the lowest scorer opens one of their envelopes and reads the dare card inside, choosing whether to live out the dare or tell their partner a 'truth'.

If you opt for the truth, keep it light. This is no time to be debating what happened at the office Christmas party five years ago; you're supposed to be having sexy fun, not provoking a row. Once you've completed the dare (or truth), turn the card over and place it face down on a table.

The highest scorer now opens one of their envelopes and repeats the above process.

Taking turns, work your way through all nine dare cards, then fit them together and, not only should you be laughing with each other, but you'll also have completed the casting board on which you'll be playing.

Once the casting board is assembled, you'll see that it's divided into four quadrants, one for each group of games. Now, one of you should hold a single die 2–5 centimetres (1–2 inches) over the 'drop zone' in the centre of the board, and release it. Whichever quadrant of the board it lands in is the section you will be picking your game from. If the die rolls off the board, try again. You can choose to play just one game or several games from that section, or roll the die onto the board again when you finish one sex game and want to try another.

Next, the other partner rolls all three dice together. Add up the total score to find your game number and turn to the appropriate page. For example, if your initial die landed in the Pleasing Him quadrant, and your roll of the three dice gave you a 1, 3 and 5, that would make your total 9, so turn to SCORE 9 in the Pleasing Him section (*page 124*). Then just follow the instructions.

GENERAL TIPS

Most of the games include a degree of physical intimacy, so only play them with someone who you're happy to get close to. Before playing, clean your teeth, have a bath and make sure that you're generally nice to be near.

If the game involves exchanging bodily fluids of any kind – oral sex or penetrative sex, for example – practise safer sex unless you have both been tested negative for sexually transmitted infections and are in a monogamous relationship. *Sex Play* is about having fun, and STIs are no fun at all.

Some of the games involve props, all of which should be found in the average household: ice, sweets, a deck of playing cards or a cup of coffee, for example. If you don't have a required prop for a game, either improvise with something that you do have in the house (using your common sense, obviously) or cast the dice again.

DEALING WITH DICELED CONFLICT

While none of the games are designed to push your limits, there is a chance that a game may instruct you to do something that you don't want to do. If this happens, don't do it! It's all very well handing your sex life over to the whim of the dice, but don't let yourself be bullied by them. *Sex Play* is about enjoying yourself, not doing things you feel uncomfortable with.

OTHER WAYS TO USE THE DICE

You can use the dice to make decisions; let's say you want to have doggie-style sex and your partner wants to have missionary-position sex; roll the dice – odds means you get your wish, evens means they get theirs.

You could make your own list of options – for example: oral sex, anal sex, vaginal sex, mutual masturbation, talking dirty and massage. Roll the dice to see which one you'll be indulging in tonight. But don't include anything on the list that both partners aren't prepared to do.

Remember: the games in this book are designed to inspire you and teach you new sex tricks to help you have more fun in bed. If you're not enjoying something, stop and move on to something else instead. Everyone is different and one person's 'winning' roll will be another's 'losing' roll. Even if you stop one activity because it's not for you, you're still teaching your partner about your desires. And you've got plenty more games to choose from. So, what are you waiting for? Get rolling ...

... Are you ready to play? ...

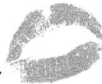

The Games

Teasers

Great sex isn't always about getting naked and squelchy. Sometimes, the sexiest thing of all can be a beguiling look, a whispered phrase or a gentle kiss. Teasers are designed to help you discover more about your partner, and to help them discover more about you. Enjoy the anticipation …

Teasers

SCORE 3

Erogenous zone Battleships

Remember playing Battleships as a child, trying to sink your opponent's ship by guessing where it was hidden? This game offers a kinky twist: you're hunting for each other's erogenous zones – on paper – instead. Get a pen and paper and prepare to find out where you should be aiming …

TO PLAY

First, each draw a grid – five boxes across and ten boxes down. Label the boxes across the top A to E and those down the side 1 to 10. Then, both of you should draw a rough figure of a person on your grid and, without showing each other, mark on the figure five crosses where your top five erogenous zones are. Each cross should fit into a single box.

Now, take it in turns to call out a grid reference to try to identify your partner's erogenous zones – for example, C6 (approximately the genitals, depending on how you draw your figure). Every time you hit a hot spot, your partner should tell you (or, to add humour, groan with pleasure). You should then ask them to elaborate on exactly where their erogenous zone is, and why. Try asking what they particularly like having done to that area: say, licking, nibbling, stroking, kissing or scratching.

Keep going until one of you finds all of the other's erogenous zones – though the other person should confess their remaining zones when they win.

BENEFITS OF THE GAME

This game encourages communication about sex, helping bridge the embarrassment gap that many people have when discussing their preferences between the sheets. It also makes both of you think about what turns you on: a surprising number of people just go with the flow and never apply thought to it.

By learning where your partner's hot spots are, you can pleasure them more effectively. No matter how long you've been together, you may learn something new; many people have unexpected erogenous zones – the backs of the knees, inner thighs or toes. Just make sure you use your new-found knowledge for good …

VARIATIONS OF THE GAME

You could mark your turn-off spots rather than your erogenous zones, as a non-confrontational way of telling your partner where you hate being touched.

You could also increase or decrease the number of erogenous zones you mark – maybe rolling one or all of the dice to decide how many you have to identify. If the dice dictate that you have to mark eighteen erogenous zones, you'll be surprised at how much it makes you think. You never know – you could discover that you have more erogenous zones than you'd ever have identified if asked directly.

And if you're happy to get naked with each other, you could award a prize to the winner: they get to have all their erogenous zones teased in the way they like most, of course.

... getting warmer ...

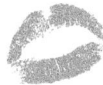

HOT TIP

Get creative when you're making your choices. Common, but less obvious, erogenous zones include:

- **The scalp** There's a lot of tension in the scalp. Washing your partner's hair can be incredibly sensual, as can softly scratching the scalp or rubbing the pads of your fingers over it.

- **Ears** Thought by some Eastern practitioners to represent the whole body (in the same way that reflexologists think the foot does); try massaging the entire ear from lobe to tip, or nibbling, sucking and blowing into the ear.

- **Creases of the body** The inner elbows, backs of the knees and crook of the neck can all be super-charged areas. Try gently trailing your nails over them, or licking them, to blow your partner away.

- **Feet** Giving a foot rub is an intimate way to show you care. Some even claim that pulling a man's toes back at the point of orgasm enhances his pleasure!

Teasers

Blank me, Baby

Sexy talk can be a fantastic form of foreplay and a
fun addition to sex, but many people feel shy about it.
This game helps you to share what turns you on in a
humorous way. After playing it, you should find it
much easier to ask for what you want.

TO PLAY

Roll a die to pick one of the words below. This word represents your primary erogenous zone:

1 = blancmange   3 = custard   5 = tyrannosaurus

2 = aardvark   4 = aubergine   6 = skoda

Now roll again to pick one of these words, to represent your secondary erogenous zone:

1 = tulip   3 = trumpet   5 = hamster

2 = caravan   4 = lollipop   6 = pogo stick

Now, complete the following sentence, picking your preferred options and using the words selected above to fill in the blanks.

'I love having my [blank] licked/sucked/stroked/bitten/ other, but my ultimate turn-on is having my [blank] licked/sucked/stroked/bitten/other.'

Your partner's role in the game is to guess which body parts your comedy words represent. Then it's their turn to roll the dice, and your turn to guess.

BENEFITS OF THE GAME

The comedy words will help you share what you want in a less intimidating way than bluntly saying it. And, if you've only recently started dating, this can also be a non-threatening way to get an idea of what your partner is into.

VARIATIONS OF THE GAME

Try writing longer stories in which to insert the comedy words. You could also make more lists of words, if two erogenous zones isn't anything like enough for you! And, of course, if you're happy to strip off with each other, you can move on to teasing the selected erogenous zones in the way requested.

HOT TIP

As a general rule, talking dirty falls into five main categories. Learn these and you'll be able to talk smut like a pro. First, there's praising a body part. For a woman, 'I love your breasts' or 'You have a gorgeous bum' can work wonders; for a man, 'You're so big/hard/big and hard' should do the trick (almost every man loves it if you praise his penis).

Then there's commending technique: 'I love the way you stroke me' or 'That was an incredible orgasm.' Don't fall into comparison though; 'That was the best orgasm I've ever had' could backfire on you by making your partner start to think about your previous lovers.

Next comes descriptive stuff: 'Do you like me trailing my hands all over you?' Don't get too flowery here; 'nipples like cherries' and 'giant man-truncheon' are best avoided (unless you want to continue the comedy).

Then there's direction-giving: 'Will you stroke my back while you slide inside me?' Make sure this doesn't sound bossy, and ideally try and throw in a comment about how much you love what your partner's doing but want more from them because they're such an incredible lover.

And, finally, there's fantasy-based stuff: 'Oh, Mr Highwayman, please don't steal my chastity.' Be careful not to go too far into your own fantasies unless you're sure your partner shares them. Otherwise it could have the opposite effect to the one you're after. Test the water first, with a mild version of your fantasy, before diving in too deeply. Similarly, don't get too cheesy or steal dialogue from adult films.

... I love the way you touch me there ...

Teasers

Look into my eyes

Attractive eyes are the second thing that a man looks for in
a woman (the first being an athletic body shape) and both
men and women find dilated pupils sexy. So use this to
your advantage. Learn how to make your pupils dilate
at will, and make your partner horny, too.

TO PLAY

Generally speaking, our pupils dilate when it's dark (to let more light in) or when we're aroused. It's one of the reasons that candle light is so romantic; the dim light means your eyes look perpetually aroused.

However, pupil dilation can be artificially stimulated. Make sure the room isn't incredibly bright or it could sting, but don't make it too dark either, or your pupils will dilate of their own accord, ruining the game you're about to play.

Kneel opposite your partner and look into their eyes. You should both rest your hands on your own thighs, and focus on breathing slowly and deeply so you're suitably relaxed. Try to breathe in time with each other, to help you build a stronger emotional connection.

There's a chance that you might start giggling. If so, don't try to fight it. Looking into someone's eyes is a very personal thing to do, and the chances are your laughter is coming from embarrassment. If you let it, out you'll either get over it or end up laughing together, neither of which is a bad outcome.

Once you're steadily gazing at each other, start thinking romantic thoughts; then dirty thoughts; then frankly outrageous thoughts. Your partner should do the same thing. After a while, you'll start to notice each other's pupils dilating.

Once you notice the pupil dilation, of course, things can start to get really interesting. You can choose to share what you were both thinking about, or you can try to maintain their dilated pupils by talking dirty and seeing what really gets them off. Even if they don't admit their fantasies, their eyes will give them away …

BENEFITS OF THE GAME

Looking into each other's eyes is a fantastic way to build a bond; by letting someone look into your eyes, you're showing that you are utterly accepting of them. And reading the body's natural arousal signs to see what turns your partner on is an erotic and interesting way to discover their sexiest secrets. As eyegazing is such an intensely personal and romantic thing to do, the chances are it will heat things up between the pair of you, too.

VARIATIONS OF THE GAME

If you're happy getting naked with each other, try caressing different parts of your own body while you look into your partner's eyes, to see what they enjoy watching the most. Team your display with softly whispered sensual words and you'll both be hot to trot in no time.

Another option is to stroke their body and see what makes their pupils dilate the most …

... Tell me your fantasies ...

HOT TIP

Emphasizing the eyes will make you look more attractive to the opposite sex. Women have it easier than men, given the vast array of make-up that's available to them – in particular, mascara and eyeliner as they can make the eyes look bigger. But men could consider investing in a pair of eyelash curlers. They may look like a medieval torture device but they're easy to use and curled lashes make the eyes look larger and more open, thus more appealing.

You can use the pupil-dilation trick when you're in public, to show your partner that you're thinking sexy thoughts about them. After all, what could be more innocent than a couple lovingly gazing into each other's eyes? Just whisper 'Look into my eyes' and start thinking all those deliciously dirty thoughts. Your partner will be desperate to get you home.

... Can you see what I'm thinking? ...

Teasers

Read my lips

Where sex is concerned, most people behave as they want their partner to

behave: men often use firmer caresses than women as they like being stroked

hard; women may use romantic gestures to show affection as that's what

they want. This game teaches you how to deliver the perfect

kiss for your partner, by following their lead.

TO PLAY

Start by blindfolding your partner, to heighten all their sensations. You don't need a proper blindfold for this: a stocking, tie or scarf will work. (If it's early in your relationship, ask your partner to close their eyes rather than blindfolding them, as covering someone's eyes demands a great deal of trust.) Tell them to relax their lips, then kiss them as you would like to be kissed.

Put your hands where you would like their hands to be when you kiss. Stick to 'safe' zones unless you are already lovers. Start as softly or as passionately as you'd like them to. Basically, deliver the kiss you've always wanted to receive.

Once you've finished, it's their turn. Remove the blindfold from them (or tell them to open their eyes). Put on the blindfold yourself, and relax while they deliver their idea of a perfect kiss. Notice any differences, such as pressure, technique or hand positioning.

BENEFITS OF THE GAME

Kissing is one of the essential elements of a relationship; according to Relate, couples that kiss regularly have more successful relationships than those who have frequent sex but don't kiss. By knowing how to deliver your partner's perfect kiss, you'll enhance every aspect of your relationship.

VARIATIONS OF THE GAME

If you're intimate with each other, this game can be used for almost any sex act, from oral sex (show a man what technique you'd like him to use by licking his palm in the right way; show a woman by sucking and licking her finger) to penetrative sex (let your partner set the pace and pick the position).

... Kiss me again ...

HOT TIP

The perfect kiss tends to start gently. Begin by touching your partner's lips with your own. Linger in the moment, enjoying the physical connection: after all, your lips are one of your most sensitive body parts. Feel the energy flowing between you and pay attention to the way your bodies feel so close together.

Don't just aim for the centre of the lips. The sides can also be sensitive, particularly if you kiss very lightly. Scatter tiny kisses over the eyelids, forehead, cheeks, nose and anywhere else that feels right.

Once the kisses are getting stronger, run your tongue softly over your partner's lips. By exploring their lips and mouth slowly, you build up a sense of anticipation, which is far sexier than shoving your tongue down their throat.

Vary your kisses to add excitement. Suck your partner's lower lip while they suck your upper lip, or suck their lower lip for a moment, lick around their inner lips, then break away to kiss them again. Some people like gentle biting – or even quite firm nibbling – so give that a go, too. Team your kisses with soft caresses of the back, hips, neck and face to heighten passion.

Remember, kissing should be sensual, so don't suck on your partner's tongue too hard – it can hurt, which is guaranteed to kill the mood. But don't be too afraid to get intense. Kissing passionately can be more arousing than direct genital contact, and some people can even climax through kissing alone.

... I'll be gentle with you! ...

Teasers

SCORE 7

Rub me the right way

The skin is the body's largest erogenous zone, so it's no wonder that massage is such a sensual treat. This game teaches you the main massage strokes you need in order to pleasure your partner. Once you've mastered the basics, your partner will be putty in your hands …

TO PLAY

Start by asking your partner to lie down on the floor or bed. They can choose to stay fully clothed or strip right off, depending on how intimate you are. If they go for the latter, make sure the heating is switched on, and cover your partner in towels so that they stay warm – goose-pimples aren't sexy.

Ask your partner to close their eyes; then roll a die to pick from the following shapes:

1 = square	3 = triangle	5 = arrow
2 = heart	4 = rectangle	6 = diamond

They have to guess the shape from your hand movements alone. Using broad, sweeping strokes (effleurage), mark out the shape on their back. Be careful not to apply too much pressure to their spine as it can be damaging, but other than that press as hard or softly as they want you to.

Once they guess the shape, roll the die again to choose one of the following letters:

1 = A	3 = T	5 = Z
2 = X	4 = S	6 = B

Ask your partner to guess the letter from your hand movements but, this time, use a kneading motion (petrissage).

Once they guess the shape, roll the die again to choose one of the following songs:

1 = Like a Virgin	4 = Leader of the Pack
2 = Lady in Red	5 = Rock around the Clock
3 = I Wanna Dance with Somebody	6 = Baby One More Time

Now, using the sides of your hands, tap out the rhythm of the song (tapotement) and ask your partner to guess what it is. Again, avoid hitting the spine.

BENEFITS OF THE GAME

By learning all the basic massage strokes, you'll be able to give your partner a truly sensual treat. In addition, the fun element will give you something to focus on other than just massaging your partner, so that you can learn how to correctly administer the strokes rather than just fixating on touching their body.

That said, make sure you pay attention to your partner's moans and groans; start gently and, if they say it hurts, stop immediately.

VARIATIONS OF THE GAME

Write a list of your own favourite songs – include 'your song' if you have one. You can also try writing sexy words and suggestions on your partner's back using massage techniques, and asking them to guess what you're writing; then see if they want to try your suggestions …

HOT TIP

Aromatherapy has been used for thousands of years, and sensual oils are referred to in books as ancient as the Kama Sutra. Some of the most aphrodisiac oils include jasmine (the scent of sacred love) rose, patchouli, ylang ylang and sandalwood. Making your own signature massage oil, by combining your favourite oils in a base of almond or peach oil, can add an erotic edge to your massage.

Warm the oil between your palms, then put both hands on the centre of your partner's back, leaving them to rest for a minute or so. This way, your partner can anticipate what's to come and get used to the feeling of your skin against theirs.

Be careful not to get any oil on your partner's most intimate areas if you're planning on having sex: oil can rot condoms, so you'll either need to share a shower or opt to use a non-oil-based lube instead.

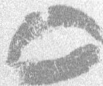

... *Please do that again* ...

Teasers

Body talking

Over 50 per cent of communication is down to body language – those
subconscious signals your body gives out when you're hot to trot. This game
helps you read each other's bodies,

and communicate your basest desires without saying a thing.

After all, sometimes actions speak louder than words.

TO PLAY

Roll a die to pick one of the following options. Don't let your partner see the list of options or what the die says.

1 = oral sex on him

2 = oral sex on her

3 = missionary-position sex

4 = woman-on-top sex

5 = doggie-style sex

6 = hand job

Now, show your partner the sex act without saying a single word. We're talking 'Dirty Charades' here. BUT, here's the tricky bit. You also have to indicate whether it's something you love, hate or don't mind either way; for example, if you are bored by the missionary position, you may want to roll your eyes while simulating it. If you love it, plaster a broad grin on your face.

Once your partner has guessed the sex act, and your feeling towards it, they have to pick their favourite sex act and simulate it for you.

And finally, you simulate your favourite sex act for them. Who knows, you may come up with an Oscar-winning performance.

BENEFITS OF THE GAME

It's relaxing, as you'll probably both end up giggling, which is always a good way to break down any barriers. It also gives you a chance to indicate your preferences in a non-judgemental way.

VARIATIONS OF THE GAME

Pick a sex act and tell your partner – but then indicate the way that you'd like it to be performed. Do you prefer missionary sex to be fast or slow? Hard or soft? With legs wrapped around each other or up in the air? By using your bodies to do the talking, you can tell each other exactly what you want.

HOT TIP

Body language isn't just something to use in the bedroom: you can employ it to signify your interest, too. These tricks will help your lover see exactly how gorgeous you find them.

- Use an 'open' posture. In layman's terms, this means making sure that your arms and legs aren't crossed, relaxing your muscles and avoiding blocking your body with any body part. Folding your arms is a big no-no.

- Touch your own body: stroke your collarbone or neck, or put your hands on your hips. This will subconsciously trigger your partner to think about touching you.

- 'Mirroring' is another way to make someone feel closer to you: copy their movements. If they lean back, you lean back; if they rest their head on their hands, you follow suit a moment or so later. This suggests, on a subconscious level, that you're similar to them.

● Leaning towards someone shows interest, as does touching their 'safe' zones: for example, brushing a piece of fluff from their shoulder or patting their leg to emphasize a point.

● 'Preening' behaviour shows keenness: flicking the hair, adjusting clothes and generally making sure that you look as good as possible.

● Looking into someone's eyes is intimate, personal and shows you feel a connection with them. So enjoy those long, languorous eye-meets. Don't stare. Just look into your partner's eyes for fractionally longer than usual, look away, then glance back. Don't worry if you feel shy and end up blushing; flushed skin is another turn-on. Your skin flushes when you have an orgasm, so blushing sends subliminal sex messages to your partner's head.

... Do it faster! ...

Teasers

Dirty Hangman

Hangman is all about filling gaps, so it's hardly surprising

that there's a sexy twist on it. This game will help you find out what turns

your partner on – and what they hate in bed. Even better, you can decide just

how wild you want things to get …

TO PLAY

First, roll a single die to choose from one of the following categories:

1 = favourite sex position	4 = favourite sex act
2 = erogenous zone	performed on a woman
3 = favourite sex act	5 = sexual fantasy
performed on a man	6 = turn-off zone

Pick a word or phrase relating to your chosen topic, and mark it out on a piece of paper with a dash to represent each letter, as per normal Hangman. For example, if you rolled a 1, you might pick missionary position. If you rolled a 5, you may choose doctors and nurses. Keep your choices simple – no more than three words. You can always elaborate further once your partner guesses the answer.

Your partner then calls out each letter: if they get one right, you add their letters in; if not, you add to your Dirty Hangman figure. The body parts drawn are: head, body, left arm, right arm, left leg, right leg and either a pair of breasts (counting as one move) or a penis.

Once your partner has guessed your phrase, it's their turn to roll the die.

BENEFITS OF THE GAME

You can communicate desires with your partner in a fun and non-threatening way – and you get to learn about their sexual mind by seeing what their guesses are.

VARIATIONS OF THE GAME

Pick something that you want to try tonight; maybe a sex position or something kinky you've always been intrigued by, like spanking. If your partner guesses it correctly, they get to take a turn and write what they'd like most tonight. If they lose, you get to live out your desire.

HOT TIP

Don't be tempted to plunge straight into your most 'out-there' desires: it's far safer to start slowly and work your way up. Say, for example, your ultimate fantasy is being chained down and whipped senseless; start with something simple, like asking your partner to pin your arms down during missionary sex (pin me down). If your favourite sex act is rimming, start with something more general like anal play so that if your partner is squeamish about the bum (as many people are) you don't scare them too much. By going in gently, you can ascertain your partner's response: after all, sex is about two people, not one.

One other word of warning: if you've been with your partner for a while and they always touch your top turn-off zone (and, if so, why haven't you told them to stop yet?), be sensitive about how you tell them – be prepared to explain exactly what it is you don't like about being touched in that particular place.

... On all fours ...

Teasers

Eat me

Experimenting with food is a fun way to tap into all five
of your senses – always a good way to enhance your sexual response. This
game requires a little preparation but will help both you and your partner to
listen to your own body, and each other's, more effectively.

TO PLAY

Ask your partner to write a list of their top four ultimate sexual or romantic desires, in order of preference. They should make sure they're all attainable given the situation you're in: so, if it's your first date, you may want to limit it to kissing or massage-level acts; if you've been together for years and get wild with each other, make sure they don't include their fantasy about you and the barmaid who works at your local! It should be something you can make true there and then – if they win.

Now, blindfold them and go into the kitchen to prepare a tray full of sensual food. Don't worry – you don't need to be a gourmet chef. Try some of the following:

- ice cubes
- slices of fruit or individual berries
- creamy liqueurs
- honey, jam or chocolate spread

Take your tray of treats through to your partner. Ask them to guess what you're feeding them (check for any allergies first so that the game doesn't backfire). Tell them to listen to the sound the food makes, if any. Can they guess what it is from sound alone? If so, they win their number-one sexual/ romantic desire. No joy? Let them smell it. If they guess correctly, they get their number-two choice. If they still can't guess, let them feel the texture with their fingers, then, if necessary, allow them to taste it. If they guess, reward them with the appropriately numbered desire on their list. If they can't guess, even after tasting it, they remove the blindfold and you get to write your list of desires, to come true if you can correctly identify the food you're given.

BENEFITS OF THE GAME

The best sex involves all five senses, so train yourself to pay attention to each of yours. Feeding someone, or allowing yourself to be fed, also enhances intimacy as it requires a degree of trust.

VARIATIONS OF THE GAME

If you enjoy cooking and have some time to prepare, go for more elaborate foods: prawns dipped in mayonnaise; smoked-salmon blinis with sour cream and chives; tiny jam tarts; or chocolate-dipped berries. Your partner must correctly identify every ingredient in order to make their sexual wish come true.

Try feeding your partner by clasping your chosen nibble between your lips for them to share with you. You may even want to sensually drizzle different wines, spirits or liqueurs from your mouth into theirs.

... Strawberries and cream? ...

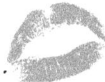

HOT TIP

Add an extra edge by including aphrodisiac foods in your tray of delights. Bananas are full of potassium, which is thought to boost libido. Oysters are full of zinc, and their shape is also suggestive, as with figs and asparagus. Honey is thought to be an aphrodisiac; the word 'honeymoon' comes from the old tradition of couples drinking honey wine on their wedding night to enhance their bedroom activities. Garlic and onions are also supposed to have arousing qualities, but make sure you cook them first unless you want to be really mean to your lover – and eat some too so you don't have to deal with their garlic breath!

And, of course, there's alcohol – but never forget what Shakespeare wrote about it enhancing desire but lessening performance: you don't want to get so drunk that you don't enjoy playing with each other.

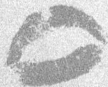

... Sense your way to a night of passion ...

Teasers

A–Z of lust

If you really want an insight into someone's sexual side, knowing the lewd thoughts and words that automatically spring to their mind can be a huge help. By using the alphabet, you can tap into their latent thoughts: after all, one person's 'dildo' is another's 'domination' …

TO PLAY

Work your way through the alphabet, taking it in turns to come up with a sex-ual word for each letter: for example, 'A' could be A-zone (the pleasure point a woman has just above her G-spot), amorous or anal sex, depending on how hard-core you want to get.

After your partner has come up with their word, you move on to the next letter – so, 'B' could stand for breasts or blow job.

The words don't have to be obviously sexual as long as you can justify why you thought of them: for example, you may go with chocolate sauce for 'C', and explain that the reason you chose it is because you love having it drizzled all over your most sensitive parts, then licked off.

If either of you fails to come up with a word, you have to roll a die and kiss an area of your partner's body, depending on which number the die falls on:

$$1 = \text{lips} \qquad 3 = \text{toe} \qquad 5 = \text{knee}$$

2 = ankle   4 = neck   6 = back

BENEFITS OF THE GAME

You'll get to learn about each other's turn-ons in a fun and light-hearted way. It'll also help you see how sexually sophisticated your partner is: if they suggest emetophilia for the letter 'E', you may want to invest in a dirty-word dictionary. If you haven't got intimate yet, the words your partner chooses will tell you how imaginative they will be in the bedroom.

VARIATIONS OF THE GAME

After each word, discuss whether it's something you love, hate or are curious to try.

Pick a sexy phrase – say, 'Make love to me now, big boy' – and come up with a sexy word relating to every letter: 'M' for masturbation; 'A' for aphrodisiac, and so on.

Alternatively, you could come up with an unsexy word for every letter of the alphabet to teach each other about your top turn-offs; say, 'N' for navel if you hate yours being touched, or 'S' for sixty-nine if you don't see the point of it. You could even throw in the names of celebs you find repulsive if you get desperate.

Or, if you have a Scrabble set, take it in turns to pick letters from a bag and come up with a dirty word beginning with that letter. As you accumulate more letters, use them to play dirty-word Scrabble.

And, obviously, you can tailor the list of places that you have to kiss if you can't guess a word, depending on how well you know each other ...

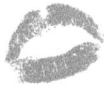

... 'E' is for 'erotic dancing' ...

HOT TIP

Everyone likes different sexual language, particularly when it comes to using it in the bedroom: one person may find harsh Anglo-Saxon terms sexier than anything else, while another might prefer more romantic words.

Don't assume that, just because you love a word, your partner will – and don't assume that women always want romantic words while men prefer baser language. It's down to personal preference rather than gender.

While you're playing this game, establish any words that either of you find a turn-off: that way, when it's time to talk dirty, you won't inadvertently use a word that makes your partner's libido shrivel. Conversely, let your partner know if there are any words or phrases that automatically make you feel frisky. By using sexual language that you both find hot, you'll enhance your lovemaking experience when you talk dirty.

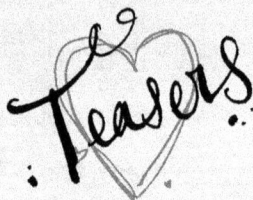

Teasers

SCORE 12

Break the habit

All too often, couples fall into a sexual rut, and not just in long-term relationships. Even after a month or so, it's common to fall into sexual habits because you know what works, and it can be easy to think 'if it ain't broke, don't fix it'. This game will help you keep things fresh.

TO PLAY

Roll a die to pick a category from the following list:

1 = date location   4 = main sexual communicator

2 = sexual position   5 = foreplay for her

3 = sexual instigator   6 = foreplay for him

Think about the category you've chosen; have you got into a habit in that area? – for example, do you always go to the cinema for dates, or are you always the person who makes the first move?

If you haven't been together long enough to form habits with each other, think about whether you, personally, have any habits. Do you tend to go for sex in the missionary position, or have you always left it to your partner to start conversations about sex?

Now, pick an alternative to your habits that you also enjoy. Resolve to avoid the activity you've got into the habit of doing, for a set period of time – say, a week, or a month. But make sure you use that time to try a variety of new things, rather than just forming another habit to replace your existing one.

BENEFITS OF THE GAME

Sexual monotony can set in very easily, and being aware of it from the early stages of a relationship will help you keep things fresh and exciting. This game will get you communicating with each other about new things you'd like to try.

VARIATIONS OF THE GAME

Change the list of topics as you see fit: maybe put in 'time we have sex' or 'day we have sex' if your sex life has become regulated. Or perhaps add 'order of sex acts' if you've got into doing the same things in the same order every time you get rampant together.

HOT TIP

If you do feel you've got into a rut, don't get angry about it: simply initiate something new. Get a sex manual to work your way through together – or simply play all the games in this book!

There's always scope to introduce something new to your sex life. Even the simplest thing, like setting the alarm half an hour early to have a morning quickie, or showering with each other at the end of the day, can help introduce variety.

One of the most common ruts that people fall into is cutting foreplay down to the bare minimum, so that both parties are merely aroused enough to be able to have penetrative sex. Try setting an alarm for 20 minutes, and put it next to the bed. Don't stop foreplay until the alarm sounds: women are much more likely to climax from penetrative sex if it is preceded by more than 20 minutes of foreplay.

... Let's try something new ...

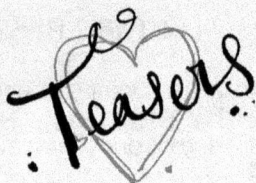

Teasers

Sexual Consequences

Remember Consequences: the game from childhood where

you created a story line by line on a folded bit of paper?

This takes the idea into more adult territory: you create your own erotic story

with your partner. Whether you decide

to make it come true is up to you …

TO PLAY

On a piece of paper, complete the first step given below. Fold the paper over so that your answer is obscured, and give it to your partner. They then complete the second step, fold the paper as you did, and give it back to you. Continue until you've worked your way through all the steps, then read the story you've created together. It could be the most erotic thing you've ever read. Then again, it might just make you laugh.

● Name a male porn star (make up a name if you don't know any).

● Write the words 'decided to try' then pick your favourite foreplay act.

● Write the word 'with' and name a female porn star (make up a name if you don't know any).

● Write the words 'in the' and add your favourite lovemaking location.

● What phrases really turn you on? Write one, followed by the words 'he gasped'.

● Now write another phrase, followed by the words 'she said. They decided on', and then add your favourite sex position.

● Add three words that describe how you most enjoy sex (for example, hard, fast).

● Write the words 'afterwards they' followed by your favourite post-coital treat.

BENEFITS OF THE GAME

This activity helps you to learn about each other's turn-ons in a fun way. Writing a sexy story together can also be an erotic experience, particularly if one of you reads it to the other when you've finished, in a sexy voice. And, even if it isn't, laughing together helps you to bond.

VARIATIONS OF THE GAME

Change the instructions to suit what you want to learn about each other; you could name the characters after yourself and your partner, start the story in your favourite date location, then cover your favourite meal, sexiest outfits, and anything else you wish before you get into more raunchy territory.

To take things to a much saucier level, set the story in a kinky location, like a dungeon, and add in lines about activities you would like to take place there – for example, spanking or bondage. The limit is set only by your imagination.

And, of course, if you really like the story, you can always live out the plot line, and even make a video of it for posterity. You don't need expensive video equipment; even a video phone will give you a high enough quality for you to enjoy watching together after you've made your story come true. Don't do this unless you know your partner very well, though: you don't want it turning up on the Internet.

HOT TIP

Writing sexy stories doesn't have to be limited to this game. Writing your lover a personalized erotic story as a surprise can be a massive turn-on, as well as showing that you think about them even when they're not around.

You don't have to be a brilliant wordsmith – you could send a story in short chunks by text message. Encourage them to respond by finishing with leading questions like 'You rip my clothes off and kiss me passionately – but what do you do next?' You'll be steaming up each other's phones in no time.

And, if you are creatively inclined, let your imagination roam free. Write a story starring your lover, with lots of references to how sexy and attractive they are. Slip it into their pocket or leave it on their pillow when you know you'll be getting home after them. By the time they've finished reading it, they'll be eagerly anticipating your arrival …

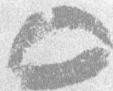

… Tell me what happens next …

Teasers

SCORE 14

Sexual spoof

Finding out what your partner really thinks about sex can be an uncomfortable subject to broach. This game helps you establish what your partner's into – handy, no matter what stage a relationship is at, as people aren't always open with each other, particularly when it comes to sex.

TO PLAY

Roll a die to pick from the following list:

1 = lingerie or nudity?	4 = adult vids or hot pics?
2 = roleplay or reality?	5 = anal sex or oral sex?
3 = foreplay or penetrative sex?	6 = dirty talk or seductive groans?

Of the two options you are given, write down the one that appeals to you most, but don't let your partner see it.

Roll the die again. If you throw an odd number, pick the first option, and for an even number pick the second. For example, if you rolled a 1 – lingerie or nudity? – followed by a 3, that gives you lingerie.

Now, talk about why this option is so much better than its alternative – in the above example you would explain why lingerie is better than nudity. Your partner must guess whether you are spoofing or telling the truth.

If you manage to spoof them, your partner has to pay a forfeit of your choice. If they get it right they take a turn, and you have to guess whether they're spoofing or not. If you get it wrong, you pay a forfeit of their choice; if not, they have to pay another forfeit for you.

BENEFITS OF THE GAME

You can find out what your partner wants in the bedroom, discover how convincing a liar they are and see how well you know them.

VARIATIONS OF THE GAME

Make your own list of options, covering any aspect of your sex life or relationship: for example, cinema or dinner date? Sub or dom? Sensual dancing or mud wrestling? Be as wild or as tame with your suggestions as you want.

HOT TIP

Communicating openly with your partner about your sexual desires can be tricky, particularly if they do something you don't really enjoy. Don't suffer in silence, but do be sensitive about the way you tell them. For example, rather than saying, 'I hate it when you touch my bum', say, 'I love the way you touch my breasts, but for some reason having my bum touched just doesn't do it for me'. That way, you're praising one of their good techniques while distancing them from the thing they do that you dislike.

Similarly, bear in mind that the bedroom isn't always the best place to raise sexual issues. It can be much less threatening to talk about things that you dislike when you're both fully clothed: say, over dinner. Being naked makes many people feel vulnerable, which is the last thing you want when you're trying to give constructive criticism about their bedroom habits.

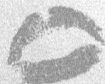

... Am I telling the truth? ...

Teasers

SCORE 15

Sexy Snap

A pack of cards can come in handy for adult games. This
one is ideal for dates early on in a relationship, as it helps
you learn more about each other – but it can easily be
spiced up if you want things to get more raunchy.

TO PLAY

Divide the cards equally between both players. Take it in turns to place a card, and, when two cards of the same number or suit are laid consecutively, the first person to shout 'snap' gets to keep all the cards that are on the table. But, the person who cries 'snap' also has to think of a way in which they and their partner are well matched: for example, both liking the same type of music, or both liking missionary-position sex.

If you can't think of anything, your partner can roll a die to choose one of the following prompts to initiate a discussion:

1 =   What are your three favourite films?

2 =   What was the first record you bought?

3 =   What's your favourite book?

4 =   Do you prefer gigs or clubs?

5 =   Would you rather have a takeaway or go to a restaurant?

6 =   Do you prefer the cinema or theatre?

Or, if you want things to get saucier, pick from the following list:

1 = What are your three favourite foreplay techniques?

2 = What was the first item of sexy clothing you bought?

3 = What's your favourite sex position?

4 = Do you prefer oral sex or hand jobs/fingering?

5 = Would you rather have sex outdoors or in the bedroom?

6 = Would you rather watch porn or go to a live sex show?

BENEFITS OF THE GAME

In the early stages of a relationship, every similarity you find seems to suggest that you're meant to be together; both parties are actively looking for reasons to be with the partner they've chosen.

As time goes on, it's easy to assume that you know everything about your partner and, therefore, stop looking for similarities, but by constantly striving to find out more about each other, you will stay as connected as you felt when you first met.

Couples with lots in common tend to have the most successful relationships. By working together to find your similarities, you'll build a bond with your partner.

VARIATIONS OF THE GAME

Make your own lists of sexy questions to ask each other. You might want to focus on one particular element of your relationship: say, foreplay or sex.

If you're already intimate with each other, you can live out each 'matching' sex act that you identify as the game progresses.

And, of course, the winner of Sexy Snap could always get the loser to pay a sexual forfeit.

HOT TIP

Don't panic if you can't think of ways in which you and your partner are similar to start with. You could well have dissimilar interests but still have a huge amount in common: for example, shared politics, religious ideas or attitude to family. These types of topics matter far more than shared hobbies: after all, in a healthy relationship, you'll see your friends regularly and can share your hobbies with them instead.

Think about the things that matter most to you in life. It may be that your work is of prime importance, or could be that your record collection is something that you couldn't imagine living without. No matter how trivial your preferences may seem, by knowing the things that are most important to you, and sharing them with your partner, you'll be giving them an insight into who you really are.

... It's great that you like that too ...

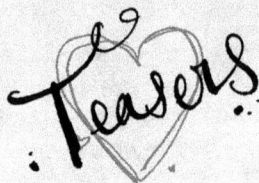

Teasers

SCORE 16

Kissing by numbers

Whoever said 'a kiss is just a kiss' was lying. Kissing can be playful, sensual,

romantic and a million and one other things. This game shows you the infinite

scope that kissing can offer

– both in the way you kiss, and where you do it …

TO PLAY

Start by rolling the die. Each number represents a different type of kiss.

1 = slowly	3 = teasingly	5 = softly
2 = passionately	4 = romantically	6 = cheekily

Now, roll again, this time to select the part of the body that you're going to kiss.

1 = lips	3 = shoulder	5 = foot
2 = neck	4 = arm	6 = back

Finally, roll a die to pick one of the following time limits:

1 = 30 seconds	3 = 2 minutes	5 = 4 minutes
2 = 1 minute	4 = 3 minutes	6 = 5 minutes

Kiss your partner in the way dictated by the die, on the body part decided by the die: for example, if you rolled a 3, a 4 and a 5, kiss your partner's arm teasingly for four minutes. Set an alarm to let you know when it's time to stop kissing.

Once you've kissed your partner's body part for the required amount of time, it's their turn to roll the die and kiss you in the manner indicated. Continue alternating rolls until you've kissed every inch of each other's bodies.

BENEFITS OF THE GAME

It can be very easy to fall into a rut, even with something as simple as kissing. This game helps you to vary your kissing techniques, and also to learn more about how your partner likes to be kissed; you may discover that they respond in a more heated manner to being kissed slowly than being kissed passionately, or that they really appreciate a cheeky nibble. Pay attention to their response, so that you can tailor your kisses accordingly in future lovemaking.

By applying the different kissing techniques to various body parts, you can also find out if your partner has any erogenous zones that you haven't yet discovered.

VARIATIONS OF THE GAME

Extend the amount of time allocated to each kiss, or write your own lists of kissing styles: for example, you may want to put 'lips only' or 'with tongue'; you may wish to add 'nibbling' or 'sucking'. Similarly, you can vary the body parts kissed – and the amount of clothing you have on while being kissed …

You could try adding an element of guesswork to the equation by not telling your partner the way that you're going to kiss them, and asking them to identify it afterwards. Reward them with a kiss in the style of their choice if they get it right.

Or, consider kissing your partner using one of the more exotic techniques detailed in the Hot Tip section that follows.

HOT TIP

Kisses don't only have to involve the lips. Butterfly kisses can be a sensual treat. To give one, simply bat your eyelashes against your partner's face or body. This feels particularly good on the most sensitive areas of the skin, like the cheeks, nipples, lower back and even genitals. It's a teasing sensation that will leave your partner wanting more.

Or, try an Eskimo kiss: rub your nose against your partner's as you look them in the eye, communicating your feelings for them visually.

Tantric practitioners suggest sharing each other's breath while looking in each other's eyes to build a connection. Be careful not to hyperventilate, though; and stop if you feel dizzy.

Another Eastern technique is exchanging saliva. Let it flow into your partner's mouth, then suck it from between their lips. They then repeat the process on you.

Get creative with your kissing techniques and you'll keep the magic in your relationship alive.

... Ooh, I like that ...

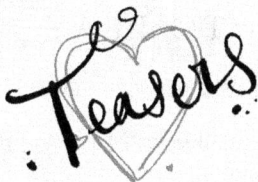

Teasers

Sexy crossword

The most important erogenous zone in the body is the brain. This game is

designed to get you thinking about sex, which,

in turn, will get you in the mood for sex. What goes on between your ears is

just as important as what goes

on between your thighs!

TO PLAY

Start by rolling all three dice. Add up your score – so, if you roll a 2, 5 and 1, your score is 8. Now, write a sexy word or phrase that has the same number of letters as your score – in this case, eight. For example, you could write 'foreplay'.

Your partner now rolls the dice and adds up their score. They then write a word with the number of letters indicated by the dice. The word should bisect yours – so, if they roll a 4, they could write 'romp' using the 'o' in 'foreplay'.

Score a point for every letter in each of your words. The winner is the person with the highest score after twelve rolls. They win a sexy forfeit of their choice.

BENEFITS OF THE GAME

Thinking sexy thoughts helps you to feel sexier. And playing this game allows you to see what's going on in your partner's sexual mind. If they write 'oral sex', 'cunnilingus' and 'tongue', you'll have a pretty fair idea of what they're most into!

VARIATIONS OF THE GAME

Take it in turns to write words or phrases – of the length indicated by the dice – that explain what you want to do tonight, each elaborating on the other's suggestions. So, you might roll a total of 10 and write 'missionary'. Your partner may follow by rolling a 12 and bisecting the 'r' of your word with the phrase 'legs in the air'. You could follow this with a roll of 13, adding 'pillow under bum' using their 'n'. Take things as far as you want to: who knows how wild your night could end up becoming?

... 'From behind' ...

HOT TIP

Don't just save your sexy thoughts for when you're with your partner. Let them know that they turn you on all the time, by sending them sexy text messages or emails throughout the day. Check their employer's email policies first, though: getting your partner the sack for receiving inappropriate emails isn't going to endear you to them. You could always ask them to set up a private email address for your kinky missives …

Let your mind wander when you're on the bus: think about the last time you made love, or an experience that you'd like to have with your partner. Keeping your sexual mind constantly engaged will help to keep your libido at a high level.

Another way to keep your mind on the erotic is to wear sexy underwear – or even nipple tassles or a rubber cock ring – underneath your normal clothes. (Don't wear a cock ring for more than an hour, as cutting off the blood supply for extended periods can be damaging.) Your sexy secret will help to keep your desires very much in the front of your mind – and make you desperate to see your partner as soon as you possibly can.

And, if you think sexy thoughts about your partner when you're pleasuring yourself, make sure you tell them about it. There are few bigger compliments that you can pay someone than admitting you've masturbated about them; though it's probably not a good idea to confess that you were thinking about their best mate joining the pair of you in bed as well …

... *Think about sex* ...

Teasers

How the other half thinks

How well do you really know your partner? Great sex isn't

an insular thing, so it's important to know what your partner's favourite things

are. This game will help you see whether you know the answers to those all-

important questions – and,

if not, it will help you learn them.

TO PLAY

To begin, each write down the following statements on a piece of paper. Leave enough space to complete each one.

1   The meal that always gets me in the mood is …

2   The song that always gets me in the mood is …

3   My favourite type of foreplay is …

4   My favourite place to have sex is …

5   My favourite way to refer to female genitals when talking dirty is …

6   My favourite way to refer to male genitals when talking dirty is …

7   My favourite way to have an orgasm is …

8   If I were to choose a sex toy to use, it would be …

9   My favourite time of day to have sex is …

10   The time of year I tend to feel sexiest is …

11   My favourite sexy item of clothing on a partner is …

12 My favourite sexy item of clothing to wear is …

13 My favourite type of afterplay is …

14 My favourite body part of my own is …

15 My favourite body part of my partner's is …

16 My favourite romantic memory from our relationship so far is …

17 My favourite sexual memory from our relationship so far is …

18 My favourite sex position is …

19 My favourite fetish is …

20 My ultimate erogenous zone is …

Both you and your partner should finish each statement – but with a twist. You should each pretend that you are your partner and guess what they'd put.

Fold the statements and put them into a container (one each). Roll a die. Whoever gets the lowest score pulls out one of their partner's answers and reveals whether they got it right or wrong. The player with the highest number of correct statements wins a sexual favour of their choice.

BENEFITS OF THE GAME

This game encourages communication between you, helping you develop your relationship. You can never learn enough about your partner's sexual preferences; it only serves to enhance your sexual experiences with each other.

VARIATIONS OF THE GAME

Tailor the statements to cover areas of weakness in your knowledge about each other; for example, you may include preferred ways to be touched or favourite fantasies.

Alternatively, if it's early in your relationship, tone the game down to include subjects like favourite places to go on a date or favourite ice-cream flavour.

HOT TIP

While learning about your partner's preferences is a healthy and useful thing to do, sometimes you may find that it raises issues in your relationship: for example, if a woman is particularly proud of her legs but her partner writes 'breasts' as his favourite body part, she may feel that he is criticizing her legs rather than praising her breasts.

Remember, this game is meant to help you discover what your partner likes about you, and how much you know about each other – and by playing it you'll enhance your knowledge of each other. So, if your partner gets all their answers wrong, don't use it as an excuse to get into a row. See it as an opportunity to teach them what you really like. You can always reinforce the message by giving them a sexy lesson in what turns you on after you finish playing …

… I feel sexiest in the spring …

Pleasing Him

It can be easy to think that men are only interested in penetrative sex and anything else is just 'trimmings', but men like being pleasured just as much as women do. These games will help you learn how to give a man the ultimate ecstasy, with your hands, lips and more …

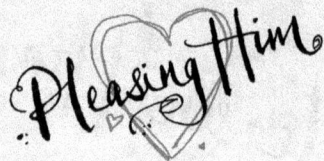

Pleasing Him

Snake charmer

Men are often a lot easier to arouse than women but, as a result, women can miss out on the subtle nuances that make the difference between a good and a great lovemaking experience. This game will help you see exactly what it is that gets your man hot.

TO PLAY

To begin, your man should be naked, while you remain fully clothed. He should be erect, too: he can either make himself hard or you can help. However, you should keep stimulation to a minimum; the fun comes later ...

Once your man is erect, roll the die to pick from:

1 = strip

2 = play with your breasts

3 = breathe over your

partner's penis

4 = talk dirty

5 = suck your finger

seductively

6 = freestyle

Follow the orders dictated by the die, watching your partner carefully to see whether his penis twitches upwards. If you roll a 6 – freestyle – do whatever you think will most arouse him. It could be an activity that's listed against one of the other scores, a combination of them or something entirely different.

The aim of the game is to make your partner's penis twitch upwards ten times within an hour. If an activity isn't having the desired effect, roll the die again and pick another activity – do this until you find something that does work. However, the golden rule is that you can't touch his penis at any point; the aim has to be achieved through visual and verbal means alone.

If you succeed in making your man's penis twitch ten times, you should be rewarded with the sexual activity of your choice. If not, he gets to choose an activity for the pair of you to indulge in.

BENEFITS OF THE GAME

When two people are busily engaged in sexual activity together, it can be easy to miss the small signs that show that the other person particularly enjoys a certain activity. By watching for your partner's physical reaction when you're not actively involved in pleasuring him, you can get an idea of what really makes him tick. This game should also reinforce the message in your own mind that pleasuring your partner is a good thing to do: after all, you get a reward if you succeed!

VARIATIONS OF THE GAME

Change the options, given to you by the die, to activities that you know your partner particularly enjoys: for example, watching you use a toy on yourself or sharing a particularly hot fantasy.

Or, if you're very sexually confident, make a list of different sexual activities and, rather than just sticking to one, your partner can roll the die every time he wants you to change what you're doing.

HOT TIP

Some women are less confident about displaying their sexual side than others. If the woman playing this game is shy, her partner should encourage her verbally as well as physically. You don't have to use words, though praising her and telling her how sexy she is will certainly help her to feel more comfortable. But moans and groans can be just as effective.

Similarly, the man may feel nervous about being so overtly on display. If this is the case, he may relax more if his partner strips off too; being the only person in a room who's naked can make even the bravest person feel vulnerable, after all. Again, moans and groans can come in handy to indicate that what's going on is doing the trick; if a woman shows how stimulated she gets when arousing her partner, it won't just be his ego that inflates …

… Now I know what makes you tick …

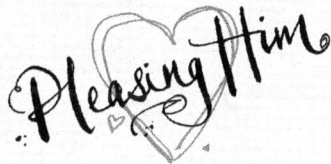

Pleasing Him

SCORE 4

The banana game

Deep-throating is a popular male fantasy, but it's not exactly the easiest thing to do, particularly if the man doesn't understand that the woman should be in control. This game will help a woman learn how to deep-throat – and teach a man how to help the woman enjoy it, too.

TO PLAY

For this game, you'll need two peeled bananas of the same size. The rules are simple. You both take your banana and, with your lips wrapped over your teeth to avoid 'grazing' the banana, you have to try to take the banana as far down your throat as you can. Make sure you use relatively firm bananas – you don't want it to break midway through and end up having a choking fit.

Take it very slowly – the aim of the game is depth rather than speed. You may find it easier if you raise your soft palate (see Hot Tip) or swallow. If you start to feel nauseous, pull the banana out and let the feeling pass before you continue.

As you get more comfortable with the banana in your throat, use your tongue to lick the underside of it, in a simulation of a blow job. Now, pull the banana out, and check it for graze marks. The winner is the person who has got the banana furthest down their throat without damaging it.

BENEFITS OF THE GAME

The woman gets to practise training her gag reflex, while the man gets to experience what deep-throating feels like and will discover why it's so important that the woman sets the pace!

VARIATIONS OF THE GAME

Use smaller or larger vegetables or pieces of fruit, to match the size of the man's member. You may even want to make a replica of his penis. You can now buy casting kits, which you can use to make a rubber clone of his most intimate part.

... I'm feeling fruity ...

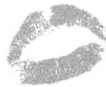

HOT TIP

The most important thing when it comes to 'deep-throating' your partner is learning how to control your gag reflex. Part of this is down to practice. However, you'll also find it a lot easier if you learn how to raise your soft palate – the soft bit at the back of your mouth. One easy way to do this is to tense your mouth, and flare your nostrils. It may not look very sexy, but you'll feel it rise, opening up your throat and making it easier for your partner's penis to slide down your throat.

The more space your throat has got, the better, so it's far easier to do with your neck straight that bent. Try lying with your head hanging off the side of the bed, and your partner leaning over you while you pull him towards your face rather than vice versa.

If your partner is too big to deep-throat – and some men are, even by the most experienced fellatrixes – use the 'cheek push'. Put one well-lubricated hand on his shaft and another on his balls. Now, position the penis so that it's aimed into the side of your cheek, while you fellate him. Let the head of his penis rub against your inner cheek with every thrust. Most men can't tell the difference in the heat of the moment; he'll feel like he's been deep-throated and your gag reflex won't be set off.

NB The golden rule with deep-throating is that the woman must be in control; the man shouldn't thrust. Instead, the woman should grip his buttocks and pull him in deeper only when she feels like she can comfortably accommodate him. If she feels her gag reflex trigger, she should simply pull back, swallow, and only resume when she feels comfortable.

... Ooh, that's a mouthful! ...

Pleasing Him

Can you feel it?

The skin is the largest erogenous zone in the body, but many couples ignore

sensual stroking, instead focusing on the 'meat of the matter'. This game

helps you to appreciate every inch

of your man's body – and, in turn, will help him tune into

his more sensual side.

TO PLAY

Each of you makes a list of your favourite sexual activities, numbering them 1 to 6. They should all be things that you could, theoretically, do tonight, so avoid anything that requires props or situations that you won't be able to accommodate, and stick to foreplay techniques and sexual positions instead.

The man then undresses and, before he lies down on the bed, you blindfold him. If your partner isn't comfortable about being blindfolded, ask him to lie on his front and close his eyes instead. Either way, make sure the heating is on; you don't want him to get cold – he's going to be there for a while.

Now, collect from around the house, six items that have a distinctive texture or sensation: a feather duster, clean tea towel, ice cube, paintbrush, suede cushion, cuddly toy or whatever you have close to hand. Don't choose anything sharp, for reasons that will become apparent as the game progresses.

Return to your partner and ask him to guess what each item is from the way it feels as you trail it over his body. Start with a relatively insensitive part of his body – say, the thick skin on his knees or elbows. If he doesn't guess, progress to the back of his hand, his inner thighs and, finally (and very gently), his genitals.

Every time he correctly identifies an object he gets a point, which can be redeemed against sexual favours at the end of the game – the first point wins him the first favour on his list, the second point wins the second favour, and so on. If he can't guess what an item is, you win a point, to be redeemed against a sexual favour on your list.

If you want to cheat, you can always strip naked and distract your partner by rubbing your body against him at the same time.

BENEFITS OF THE GAME

The man will have to pay far more attention to the signals his body sends him than he would usually; the blindfold will help with this by heightening his remaining senses.

And, depending on how sensually you trail the objects over his body, this game can also double as foreplay …

VARIATIONS OF THE GAME

Rather than using items from around the house, you could use different parts of your body – say, your hair, nails, teeth, nipples, pubic hair and feet. Your partner has to guess which part of your body you are using to caress him.

If you want to make the game more difficult for him, you can set a time limit in which he has to identify the object or body part.

HOT TIP

Don't just save sexual experimentation like this for playing dice games. Use different textures to add sensation to your usual lovemaking. Try stroking your partner while wearing a leather, lace, lambs-wool or latex glove. You can also get feather ticklers and suede ribbons that are specifically designed for sex play.

Run an ice cube over his buttocks, or trail a feather down his spine while you make love. In particular, run it over his coccyx – the small dimple in the base of his spine, which Tantric practitioners believe to be the sexual centre.

Tease your nails sensually over his back – but don't scratch hard unless you know he likes it. Or let your hair run over his balls when you're performing a blow job. By varying the ways you touch your partner – and the things you touch him with – you'll add a new dimension to your lovemaking.

... *That tickles!* ...

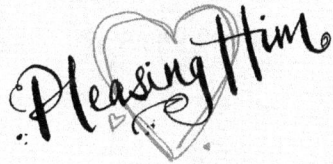

Pleasing Him

SCORE 6

Strip dice

All too often, couples just rip off their clothes and get down

to it, missing out on the erotic treat of slowly undressing each other. This

game helps bring back the anticipation of peeling off your clothes slowly –

but with a twist. You aren't

allowed to use your hands …

TO PLAY

Write a list of six articles of clothing that your partner is wearing, and number each one. For example:

$$1 = \text{trousers} \qquad 4 = \text{socks}$$
$$2 = \text{underwear} \qquad 5 = \text{tie}$$
$$3 = \text{shirt} \qquad 6 = \text{jumper}$$

If he is wearing less than six pieces of clothing, count each sock as an individual item and, if that still doesn't give you enough options, include an item more than once.

Now, the man rolls a die. You then remove the article of clothing that corresponds to his throw – but without using your hands. You can use your lips, teeth (careful about taking his underwear off with them!), elbows, feet or any other part of your body. If there is clothing on top of the item you're trying to remove, you'll have to get that out of the way first.

If you fail to take off the chosen item of clothing in an agreed amount of time – say, 10 minutes – you have to pay a sexual forfeit.

BENEFITS OF THE GAME

By taking your time removing your partner's clothes, you'll get to study his body a lot more closely than usual. He may well find it a turn-on having you remove his underwear with your lips. Or, you could just end up laughing together, which is always a great way to build a bond between two people.

VARIATIONS OF THE GAME

If you want to be really strict – and you totally trust each other – the man can tie the woman's hands together. Or, if he wants to get you naked too, you could take it in turns to roll the die and remove an item of each other's clothing.

HOT TIP

When you're next embarking on a sexy night, rather than rushing to remove your partner's clothes, take your time. Caress his chest and nipples as you slowly unbutton his shirt. Kiss each inch of naked skin that you uncover. Tease his back with your fingertips when you slip his shirt off.

As you progress further down, rub his penis through his trousers for a while before you slo–o–o–wly peel down his zip or pop the buttons on his fly. Slip your hand inside and caress his penis before pulling your hand away and trailing your nails gently over his inner thighs.

Give him a foot massage after you remove his socks, and kiss his legs once you pull his trousers from him. Work your way, agonizingly slowly, up his body and breathe on his penis through his underwear before you remove that final item of clothing. After all, the best things come to those who wait ...

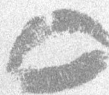

... Take it slowly ...

Pleasing Him

SCORE 7

Look, no hands

It can be easy to settle into lovemaking routines. This game helps you avoid the

old ruts by making you think of new

and unusual ways to pleasure your partner. Not only are

the sensations very different, but the techniques are also

handy alternatives if you get tired during more

conventional methods.

TO PLAY

Start by rolling a die to select one of the following options:

1 = crook of elbow	4 = between buttocks
2 = feet	5 = between thighs
3 = between wrists	6 = armpit

Now, stimulate your man using that part of your body alone, until he reaches climax. If the option you've chosen just isn't doing the trick or you get too tired using one body part, roll the die again to choose another one.

Bear in mind that if you roll a 4 or a 5, you should make sure that the man wears a condom unless you've both been tested for STIs and are protected against pregnancy; the head of the penis has over 3 million sperm on it so it's not worth taking any risks. And, if you roll a 2, check that the skin on your feet isn't too rough as you don't want to snag your man's most delicate skin.

BENEFITS OF THE GAME

By learning how to stimulate your partner with every inch of your body, you'll add variety to your lovemaking. Different body parts give very different sensations, too. And, you'll have new alternatives to fall back on if your wrist gets tired when stimulating a man with your hand.

VARIATIONS OF THE GAME

Make your own list of body parts with which to stimulate your partner: your hair, between your breasts or anywhere else you can imagine.

You'll find this game much easier, and more pleasurable, if you use lubricant to help things slide more easily. Don't use an oil-based lube if you're planning sex later, though, as these can rot condoms.

HOT TIP

Don't think that the woman always has to be the one to move when stimulating a partner. The advantage of using a lubricant is that it allows a man to slide easily, meaning that the woman can lie back while the man thrusts, setting his own pace and rhythm.

To masturbate a man with the crook of your elbow, simply lube it up, bend your arm and sit down while he stands next to you and thrusts. If you're using your feet, try lying on your back and touching the soles of your feet together, leaving a gap in between your arches for him to thrust between. With your wrists, just move your arms up and down; and between the buttocks, simply lie face down and let him grind against you while you thrust your buttocks back. Use a similar technique to masturbate a man between your thighs; and finally, if using your armpit, sit on a chair with your arm at your side while the man stands next to you and thrusts his penis into it.

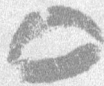

... Rub against me ...

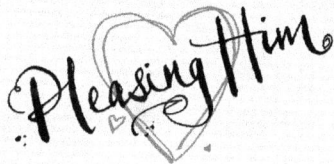

Pleasing Him

SCORE 8

Oral pleasures

Oral sex is incredibly popular with many men, but women often rely on just one technique. This game will teach you new ways to pleasure a man with your mouth and, in doing so, introduce variety to your lovemaking experience. Just make sure you pay attention to the techniques he really loves.

TO PLAY

Pick from one of the following techniques by rolling one of the dice.

1 = deep throat. See the Hot Tips section of The Banana Game (pages 104–5).

2 = fire and ice. This is way less scary than it sounds. You will need to have to hand a hot drink and some ice cubes. Alternate taking a mouthful of warm (not boiling) liquid and sucking your partner, with sucking an ice cube while you fellate him.

3 = humming. Simply hum while you give your partner a blow job. The vibrations will add an extra edge for him.

4 = sword swallower. Use your hands as well as your mouth. Get your palm wet with saliva or flavoured lubricant so that he can barely tell where your hand ends and your mouth starts, and fire his penis into your cheek. He'll feel like you're deep-throating him.

5 = lip service. Give him more of a teasing experience, using only your lips to pleasure him. But don't just kiss him. Let the underside of your lower lip run over his frenulum – the stringy bit on the underside of the head of his penis. Use your lips to gently nibble up his shaft and breathe onto his balls with your lips pressed against them.

6 = suction. Slowly suck his penis into your mouth, feeling it harden, but rather than using your tongue to tease him just suck harder the more aroused he becomes. Don't suck so hard that it hurts him, though!

Set an alarm clock for 2 minutes. Now, perform a blow job on your partner using the method suggested by the die, until the alarm goes off. Then, roll the die again and try another technique.

BENEFITS OF THE GAME

By working your way through all the options, you'll add to your blow-job skills and techniques. Any that he particularly enjoys can then be added to your normal lovemaking.

VARIATIONS OF THE GAME

Make your own list of blow-job styles, based on what your partner likes. For example, if he has sensitive testicles, add in some options that just stimulate them. If he likes a more aggressive approach, add in nibbling. And, if he likes a gentle touch, add lapping or even just blowing; although it isn't how the blow job got its name, seductively blowing over the penis and testicles can be a sensual treat.

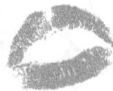

... You blow me away ...

HOT TIP

If you're not particularly keen on giving blow jobs, your man can do a lot to help himself. To start with, he can ensure that he washes regularly to avoid build-up of smegma and generally nasty niffs. Drinking pineapple juice makes semen taste sweeter, as does avoiding cigarettes, alcohol and spicy foods.

And, if you don't like swallowing, or haven't been tested for STIs, add a flavoured condom to the equation: it gets rid of any panic that a man may not be able to hold himself back.

You may also want to incorporate food into giving blow jobs: chocolate sauce drizzled over the penis and slowly licked off can make it a sweeter experience for the woman – and a decadent treat for the man.

Similarly, champagne or sparkling wine can be used to good effect during oral sex: the bubbles bursting on the man's penis add extra zing, while the woman gets to enjoy a mouthful of her favourite tipple at the same time as enjoying a mouthful of her man!

Pleasing Him

My favourite thing

All too often, couples rely on guesswork to determine what each other likes.

While exploring one another's bodies is all very well, a bit of direction can go

a long way. This game teaches you about your partner's ultimate turn-on –

and you get to have fun finding out what it is …

TO PLAY

The man starts by rolling a die to choose from the following options:

1 = fellatio technique	4 = sexual position
2 = hand-job technique	5 = fantasy
3 = sexy outfit for your partner to wear	6 = body part to be stimulated (excluding penis)

He then writes down his favourite thing in the category he has selected: say, being sucked slowly from flaccidity to full erection, or making love with you on top.

You then have to guess what he has chosen, either by asking or by demonstrating what you think his answer will be. He says 'hotter' or 'colder' to indicate how close you're getting to the option that he's written down.

Your partner should be as specific as possible when writing down his options: the more detail he goes into, the longer the game will take and the more fun you'll both have. It also means that you will get to learn more about exactly what it is that really turns your man on.

BENEFITS OF THE GAME

If the man goes into detail about the things he most enjoys in the bedroom, you will learn how best to please him when you're getting intimate. And, by playing a game rather than simply having a conversation, it's less confrontational and much easier for both of you.

VARIATIONS OF THE GAME

Rather than using a die to pick from the options, start with an 'open brief': you have no clues as to what type of activity your partner has written down and have to, instead, work through your sexual repertoire to see what your partner likes the most. Be warned – this may take some time ...

HOT TIP

Many people make the mistake of assuming that their partner will enjoy a particular activity just because their previous partner did. Everyone is different, so you shouldn't be surprised if a sure-fire hit with one partner is an utter flop with another.

If you've only recently met your partner, spend time in the early days of your relationship learning about each other's bodies and turn-ons. It's much easier to discuss this when you first meet, before either of you have worked through your repertoire of sex moves, as it feels less judgemental; it's not a case of what your partner's done wrong in the past, but simply a case of what you respond to best.

Don't panic if you've been together for a while, but have never discussed these issues: now is your chance. And by far the easiest way to share what you most enjoy is to show each other. To start with, masturbate in front of each other. As you progress, move your partner's hand on top of yours to show them the level of pressure and speed that you're using to get yourself off. A woman may find it easiest to hold her partner's hand by the wrist and guide him, taking control of the level of pressure that he applies, while a man may find it easiest to put his hand over the top of his partner's and move her hand as he'd move his own.

There's no need to be embarrassed about sharing what you like, or masturbating in front of each other: after all, if you know each other well enough to have sex, you know each other well enough to say what you like best.

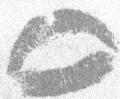

... You're getting hotter! ...

Pleasing Him

SCORE 10

You've got rhythm

Different strokes for different folks, or so the old saying goes. But it's surprising how many people don't bother to vary the rhythm when they're performing sex acts, instead using the same speed with every partner. This game helps you find out how fast or slow your partner really wants to go.

TO PLAY

Pick six songs that you like, and that are easily accessible. They should each have a different tempo: say, a romantic ballad, a fast dance number, a classical piece, and whatever else you're into.

Write down the song titles, numbering them from 1 to 6. Now, roll a die to choose a song. Throw again to pick one of the following sex acts:

1–2 = hand job

3–4 = blow job

5–6 = penetrative sex

You have to perform the sex act indicated in time to the chosen song. Remember, this game is designed with the man's pleasure in mind, so the woman takes control: the man simply lies back and enjoys himself. If a certain song isn't working, roll the die again and select another song.

BENEFITS OF THE GAME

By varying the rhythm with which you perform sex acts, you change the sensation: fast sex is often deeper, too, whereas slow sex can be more sensual. A romantic tune will give you time to deliver a lingering blow job, while a dance number may be better suited to deeper thrusting. Most people tend to use a consistent rhythm when they make love and, therefore, miss out on the infinite pleasures afforded by ringing the changes.

VARIATIONS OF THE GAME

Put the radio or music television on instead, and vary the pace of your lovemaking to fit with each new song that comes on. Or, if you don't have a stereo or television in the bedroom, imagine the song going through your head – or get your partner to sing to you, if you're sure it won't ruin his concentration!

HOT TIP

The faster you move during sex – be it penetrative or otherwise – the greater the need for lube. After all, speed equals friction and too much friction can be painful.

Experiment with the way you apply lube, to offer a sensual treat. Drizzle it over your partner's penis from a few inches above, so that he gets a shocking sensation. Or, fill your navel with lube and get your partner to slowly run his penis backwards and forwards through it until he's suitably lubricated. This trick also works well between a woman's breasts. Make applying lube part of your lovemaking rather than just a necessary, but boring, task.

... Build the heat with the beat ...

Pleasing Him

SCORE 11

Handy hints

There are numerous different ways to pleasure a man using your hands, but

lots of women rely solely on the old 'up

and down' motion. This game helps you to explore the

various different techniques, to see which one will

make your man melt the most.

TO PLAY

Start by rolling a die to choose from one of the following options:

1 = basket weaving. This is Lou Paget's classic technique. Link your fingers together and clasp both hands around the shaft of your partner's penis. Push your hands to the base of the shaft and twist them. Then slide your hands to the top, twist them over the head of the penis, and repeat.

2 = making fire. This has nothing to do with matches! Put one hand on either side of your partner's penis, and then rub it between your hands as though you're using a stick to start a fire.

3 = the birdcage. This is a simple technique that will stimulate his entire length. Just grip the shaft with one hand while you stroke the head of his penis with the other, rotating it for maximum pleasure.

4 = the rings. Simply form two 'OK' signs with your hands, and place them both around the head of your partner's penis. Move them up and down the shaft, keeping up a steady motion and speed as your partner gets more aroused. When your fingers reach the top of the penis, twist the rings in opposite directions to each other, to add an extra thrill.

5 = the rope. Use both hands alternately to caress your partner, as though you're letting out a thick, endless rope. Each time you reach the top of the penis, let your thumb rub over the frenulum – the 'stringy bit' under the head of the penis – as many men find this area particularly sensitive.

6 = the heartbeat. Clasp your hands together, as for 'basket weaving', opposite. Then 'pulse' them as you slide them up and down his penis. This mimics the way your vagina moves around him.

Now, give your partner a hand job using the technique suggested by the die. Make sure you have lots of lubricant to hand, as all the techniques are far more pleasurable if performed on a lubed penis.

BENEFITS OF THE GAME

By varying the way you caress your partner, you may well find a technique that gets him to 'blast off' more effectively than the 'up-and-down' motion – or, at least, gives him extra pleasure.

VARIATIONS OF THE GAME

Buy one of Lou Paget's books and choose from her many masturbation techniques.

... *You haven't done it like that before!* ...

HOT TIP

Two hands are better than one, or so the old saying goes, and nowhere is this more true than with hand jobs. Using two hands allows you to stimulate your partner in more ways – say, stroking the head while pumping his shaft. It also means that you're less likely to get tired quickly as you can alternate the hand that is 'taking the strain'.

Using one hand to slide up towards the head of the penis while the other slides down to the base of the penis can give an interesting 'stretching' sensation, while tickling the balls or tugging on them at the point of orgasm can also add an extra thrill. Check first, though, as some men's testicles are too sensitive to be touched.

During masturbation, you can also try caressing the perineum: the area between the base of a man's penis and his anus. By pressing firmly, you can even stimulate the male G-spot from the outside: ideal if he's too squeamish to let you go for direct prostate stimulation.

Pleasing Him

Ball girl

The testicles can be incredibly sensitive, but it's amazing how often they're ignored in lovemaking. By learning how to caress a man's testicles in the right way for him, you'll add a new dimension to your lovemaking and, if you have a man's balls in your hand, his heart will surely follow!

TO PLAY

Start by rolling a die to pick from one of the following options:

1 = teabagging. This involves lying underneath the man while he kneels above
your face and lowers his scrotum into your mouth (in the same manner as a
teabag is lowered into a cup of hot water, hence the name). Suck each testicle
into your mouth, then try sucking both into your mouth at the same time, if
you can do so without grazing him with your teeth. Lick him while you're sucking his balls; and, for a double thrill, stroke the shaft of his penis as well.

2 = bobbing for apples. Lie underneath your partner with him kneeling astride
your face but, rather than letting him take control and lower his testicles into
your mouth, start by licking the underside of his testicles, then gradually move
your neck upwards so that you can take each testicle into your mouth in turn.

Sucking the skin in between the testicles can also give him pleasure – it can take slightly harsher treatment, so you may want to softly nibble it.

3 = Chinese balls. Take his scrotum very gently in your hand and roll his balls in your palm. DON'T squeeze unless he asks you to: testicles are very easily bruised.

4 = breath of fresh air. This means you simply breathe all over his testicles; get close so that he can feel the heat of your breath.

5 = tug and tease. Cup his testicles in your hand while you stroke his shaft and, as he nears orgasm, gently pull them downwards.

6 = tickling. Simply tickle the testicles softly. You can add an interesting sensation by pressing the heel of your hand into your partner's perineum (the area between the base of the penis and the anus) with one hand while the other tickles his balls.

Pleasure your partner in the manner indicated by the die. If you feel like trying a different technique, roll the die again.

BENEFITS OF THE GAME

The testicles are often ignored during foreplay and sex, but stimulating them can make a real difference to your lovemaking. It also helps build a bond between you and your partner: after all, he's showing immense trust by letting you hold his balls in your hand.

VARIATIONS OF THE GAME

Buy a sex manual with more ball-play techniques, and make your own list of options. Don't just think about using your hands and mouth: consider stroking them with a silk scarf, a feather or fake fur.

... Let's play ball! ...

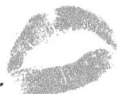

HOT TIP

Don't just tease the testicles during foreplay. Move your hand down between your legs during sex to caress your partner's balls while you make love. Combine this with pressing the heel of your hand into his perineum as above, and he'll probably come much quicker than usual!

You can also use a vibrator to stroke a man's balls during sex (or any other act), to add extra sensation. It may be too ticklish to start with, so don't switch the vibrator onto maximum rev straight away: start slowly and work your way up.

Tugging on the balls at the point of orgasm is thought to enhance the sensation for many men. This is easiest done in the missionary position, or by reaching between your legs during doggie-style sex. Be careful not to press too hard, though; this isn't the time to start experimenting with a man's pain/pleasure threshold.

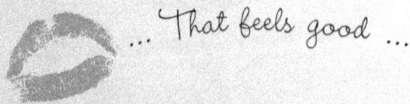

... That feels good ...

Pleasing Him

Sweet surprise

The longer foreplay lasts, the more intense a man's orgasm
will be. This game will take him to the very limits of his endurance – but the
end result will definitely be worth it. Anyway, how much is he really going to
complain about being stroked all over?

TO PLAY

The sweet shop may seem like a strange place to go to improve your sex life, but you'd be surprised at how much fun penny sweets can be for adults. Start by rolling a single die to establish which sweet you're going to play with.

1 Sherbert Dip The fizz makes oral sex extra-special – but careful where you put the dipper …

2 Space Dust Imagine the sensation of it popping over your most sensitive parts – or even sharing a kiss and feeling it pop together.

3 Liquorice bootlace To tie each other up, then nibble away.

4 Mars Bar With the number of stories about them, sex play with a Mars Bar has to be tried at least once!

5 A Finger of Fudge Like a Mars Bar, but smaller, leaving more options open.

6 A packet of Extra Strong Mints Makes your bits tingle as well as giving you
   minty-fresh breath.

Once you've picked your sweet, the fun can start. You have to wait outside the
bedroom, or close your eyes, while your man hides the sweet somewhere on
his body; he could tuck it into an article of clothing, or he may decide to get
somewhat racier …

   Now, roll all three dice and add the throws together to get a total score. Then,
follow the instructions below. The woman's mission, in all cases, is to find the sweet.

3–6 Women Search for the hidden sweet, but without using your hands; you
could use your lips, tongue, elbows and even your feet to search every inch of
your partner's body. While it can be tempting for the man to just lie back and

enjoy the sensation, this game offers a great opportunity for communication. If you touch your man in a way that he particularly likes, he should tell you. That way, it can be incorporated into your sex play on a regular basis.

7–12 Men Use chocolate body paint or honey drizzled over your body to lead your partner to the place where you've hidden the sweet. But, she has to lick every bit of it off before she's allowed her reward.

13–18 Women Blindfold your man, then breathe all over his body. He should say 'warmer' or 'colder' as you move closer to, or further away from, the sweet. Every time you get 'warmer', you can get more intimate: start using your tongue and lips to search, or trail your fingers softly over his body. The blindfold will heighten the sensation for the man.

BENEFITS OF THE GAME

The man gets teased all over and the woman gets to learn about his erogenous zones.

VARIATIONS OF THE GAME

Skip the first step and use sweets you already have in the house, but bear in mind that chocolates will get you particularly sticky – go for a boiled sweet instead if you're really concerned about the sheets. But, come on: good sex is about getting sticky together …

… Get sticky with me …

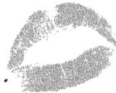

HOT TIP

Playing with food can be fun but make sure you wash thoroughly afterwards: sugar can encourage thrush in women, which isn't likely to make for a sensual mood.

But, don't just dash off to the bathroom when you've finished playing. Think about trying some classic role-play – naughty nurse and patient. Administer a bed bath with warm, soapy water, paying particular attention to the genitals, of course. Use a flannel and a sponge to give alternating sensations and squeeze water so that it runs erotically over the man's penis and perineum. Put towels down first, though: you don't want a wet patch the same size as the bed.

If you want to get really kinky, you can even add a nurse's uniform: either bought from a sex shop or home-made from a white dress teamed with a children's toy first-aid kit.

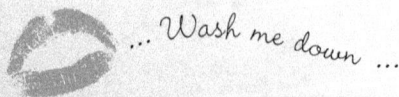

... Wash me down ...

Pleasing Him

SCORE 14

Strip cards

This is a classic game but, this time, with a twist. If the man loses a hand he

has to remove his clothes, but (rather than

just stripping off too) the woman has to pay a forfeit.

This is one game that can get really steamy …

TO PLAY

Use a standard pack of playing cards and deal each person two cards. Add up your score from the two cards – an ace can equate to 1 or 11 and picture cards are worth 10. The aim of the game is to score 21. Take it in turns to decide whether to add another card (twist) or stay with the cards you have (stick). Whoever scores closest to 21 without going over, once you have both decided to stick, wins the hand.

If the man loses the hand, he has to remove an item of clothing. If the woman loses a hand, she also has to remove an item of clothing – and pay a sexual forfeit of the man's choice ... All forfeits should last no longer than 2 minutes – set an alarm to make sure you stick to the time allocation, as it prolongs the teasing.

The game continues until you've used all the cards in the pack – or until neither of you can resist taking things further.

BENEFITS OF THE GAME

This game makes foreplay last for ages: because of the stop/start nature of the teasing, it will keep taking a man to the edge, then back down again. This will massively intensify his eventual orgasm.

The game will also show you exactly what your man wants – and how mean he is when it comes to choosing forfeits …

VARIATIONS OF THE GAME

You can add a stripping and forfeit element to any game of cards. Pick your favourite game to play. Or, if cards aren't your thing (or you don't have a deck to hand), try it with other quick games, like Noughts and Crosses.

… Take off all your clothes …

HOT TIP

If you're going for a gambling theme, why not indulge in a James Bond/ Bond girl scenario. This can be arousing for both of you, as it taps into a primal desire for a man to be dominant and a woman to be 'taken'.

Set the scene if you can: dim the lights, light candles, burn incense and generally turn your bedroom into a Bond-style seduction pad. Get dressed up to play cards. The man could wear a tuxedo (real bow-ties are much sexier than pre-tied ones) and sip a Martini. The woman could wear a glamorous bikini and adopt a suggestive name like 'Ivana Man'.

Get into character to fully indulge the fantasy. Maybe the woman is a secret agent who has to search James Bond's body for hidden spy equipment. Or perhaps he'll over-power her and tie her up in order to make his escape – but not before taking full advantage of her vulnerable position. Sex toys can double as the very latest gadgets from MI5!

You may feel silly at first, but if you let your imagination run free it's amazing how quickly you can get into it. And, stepping outside your normal roles can help you experiment with new lovemaking techniques – after all, James Bond is a master of seduction, isn't he?

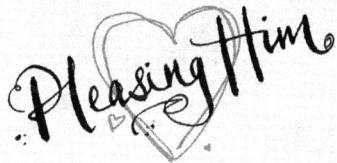

Pleasing Him

SCORE 15

Body painting

Think you know exactly how your man wants to be touched? Are you

prepared to put it to the test? This game helps you

see exactly how well you know your partner. And he

gets to enjoy the erotic sensation of a paintbrush

tickling his most sensitive parts …

TO PLAY

For this game, surprisingly enough, you'll need body paints. You can get paint specially designed for body painting or just use children's face-painting crayons. The former is preferable as they're applied with a brush, which is much more sensual than a crayon.

Your man starts by drawing a picture of his body, without you seeing it. He then labels each body part with the act that he most likes having performed on it: for example, he could write 'suck' next to his penis or 'massage' next to his shoulders.

Once your partner has finished labelling his picture, he puts it into an envelope, and then strips naked – make sure the room is warm as he'll be naked for a while and you don't want him to get goose-bumps. You then begin to paint on his body. But, rather than just drawing pictures on him, you paint words specifying what you think he most likes having done to that body part: for example, you could paint the word 'nibble' on his thighs, or 'kiss' over his lips.

Once you have completed your masterpiece, your man opens his envelope and you compare your guesses with his answers. You get a point for every answer you get right, to be redeemed against sexual favours.

BENEFITS OF THE GAME

Not only does this game help you learn about what your partner most wants done to his body, but the sensation of the brush or paints will give him a sensual thrill.

VARIATIONS OF THE GAME

If you don't have any body paints, you can just use lipstick or eyeliner to paint your partner's body.

HOT TIP

Paintbrushes aren't just useful for this game; a set of clean, dry paintbrushes from your local DIY store make for a cheap and frivolous sex aid. Get the softest ones you can (unless you're into pain) and use them to stroke sensually over your partner's body. Team with a set of make-up brushes for more precise and softer stroking.

A paint roller can also be used in an erotic way. Get your partner to lie down, naked, on a towel as if you were going to give them a massage. Straddle them and use the roller to run up and down their back: it's a cheap alternative to massage rollers. Hard, plastic paint rollers can be used to work out muscular tension, while foam rollers can be soaked in massage oil to get your partner oiled up all over. Whichever type you use, make sure you avoid pressing on the spine as it can be dangerous.

Once your partner is feeling suitably relaxed, ask them to turn over, and run the paint roller up their legs and over their inner thighs. With a make-up brush in your other hand – an eyeliner brush is ideal – tease their genitals: run it over a woman's clitoris and labia, or trail it over the vein running up a man's penis.

A blusher brush can be used to dust your lover with sweet-tasting body dust, which you then lick off. There are various flavours available in the shops, but if you don't have any to hand, sherbet or even icing sugar will make a serviceable alternative.

After you've brushed your partner all over, they'll be dying for you to brush your body against theirs …

… You are a work of art …

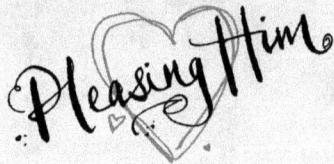

Pleasing Him

The memory game

Remember the game where you place items on a tray, ask someone to

memorize them, then remove one and see if they

can remember what you've removed? This game adds a sexy

twist – and you can guarantee that your partner's memory

will improve when he sees what you do with the items …

TO PLAY

Start by filling a tray with at least ten sexy items. They don't all have to be obviously designed for sex: you could include things like a jar of honey for drizzling over your partner's genitals, or a silk scarf to run sensually over his body. Other items could include a sex toy, a pair of handcuffs or a tie for bondage fun, a feather, a bottle of lubricant, a condom, an erotic book or sexy video; anything that you can use in your sex play.

Now, give your partner a minute to memorize all of the items on the tray. Ask him to turn away or close his eyes at the end of the minute, then remove one of the items and place it out of view. He now has to guess which item is missing. If he guesses it correctly, he wins a sexual favour of his choice. But, if he loses, things get really interesting ...

Put the missing item back on the tray, and then give a demonstration of exactly how each item can be used in your sex play: for example, run the feather over his testicles, give him a brief taste of a hand job with the lubricant or put the condom on him with your mouth. Work your way through all ten items, giving him only a brief taster of the joy that they can give him. Once you've demonstrated all ten items, and he's desperate with anticipation, tell him to close his eyes again and remove one of the items. After you've shown him exactly what you can do with each item, you can guarantee he'll find it a lot easier to remember. And, he'll be more than anxious to win his sexual favour …

BENEFITS OF THE GAME

Not only do you get to experiment with lots of fun accessories; this game will also help your partner to form kinky mental associations with all the items on the tray – he'll smile every time he puts his tie on in the morning!

VARIATIONS OF THE GAME

To make the game easier or harder, vary the number of items you use, or the amount of time you give your partner to memorize them.

Or, write down different sex acts on a piece of paper and get him to memorize those instead – and demonstrate them all, if need be. You could make him pay you a sexual forfeit if he can't guess the item, before you go on to prompt his memory.

... How good is your memory? ...

HOT TIP

Once you start thinking about things in a sexual way, it's amazing how many alternative uses for common household items you'll find.

A clothes peg can double as a nipple clamp (but use the plastic ones rather than the wooden ones if you're not that pain-driven, as they're less tightly sprung).

Bubble bath and water can be used to give a Thai massage, in which the woman lies on top of the man, naked, and writhes against him letting the foam slide erotically between you.

A candle can be used as a substitute dildo (but make sure it's white rather than coloured, as the dye can come off otherwise).

Do make sure that you use your common sense: use a condom over anything inserted into the vagina or anus to protect against germs, and never insert anything that isn't easily removable. The golden rule is, if in doubt, don't.

... Where have you hidden the feather? ...

Pleasing Him

SCORE 17

Just desserts

Chocoholic girls are going to love this game! Food can be a sensual addition to sex. Through smothering your man in your favourite sweet treats and eating them off him, you'll learn where he most likes to be licked and, in the meantime, you get to enjoy your just desserts …

TO PLAY

This game takes a bit of planning but it's worth it. Start by going shopping for all your favourite sweet treats: ice-cream, whipped cream, mousse, fresh fruit, chocolate sauce and anything else that takes your fancy,

Now, put a plastic sheet or a cut-open bin bag on the floor. Get your partner to lie down on it and create the dessert of your dreams on his naked torso. Treat this as fore-play: drizzle chocolate sauce slowly over his thighs, and pour whipped cream over his penis while you hold and stroke it, or put chocolate buttons, strawberries or cherries on his nipples, rolling them around as you do so to stimulate him. Try peeling a grape and running it up his shaft before circling the head of his penis with it.

Once you've got your partner suitably smothered in all your favourite desserts, lick, suck and nibble them off. You are both likely to get very messy – but that's half the fun of the game. And, if you get too sticky, he can always clean you up with his tongue.

BENEFITS OF THE GAME

He is given lots of foreplay while you get to enjoy your favourite dessert, although there's nothing to stop you from feeding him food while you decorate him – or letting him take food from your lips as you nibble it off.

VARIATIONS OF THE GAME

Get your partner to lie in the bath rather than on a plastic sheet while you decorate him – then get in there and start eating, before filling the bath up to clean each other off.

And, if you don't have a sweet tooth, use savoury food like cheese spread from a tube, olives and cucumber instead. Avoid anything spicy, though – it can sting and cause irritation.

HOT TIP

This game gives you a chance to explore your partner's body with your lips and tongue, so pay attention to the way he responds to each nibble, lick and bite and you'll learn techniques that can be incorporated into your day-to-day love-making. Ways to pleasure a man with your lips and tongue include:

Foot-sucking Take one or more of his toes in your mouth and suck on them, varying the suction from light to hard. Reflexologists believe that each part of the foot corresponds to a different part of the body. The big toe relates to the head, while the genitals are represented about halfway down the sole. If your man's got ticklish feet, use firm pressure with your fingers to desensitize him, then move on to licking.

Nipple-nibbling Men's nipples can be just as sensitive as women's but are often ignored. Swirl your tongue around his nipple, and gently nip it with your teeth or suck it between your lips. Tease his other nipple with your fingers at the same time.

Rimming Not for the faint-hearted, but some couples really enjoy rimming – licking the anus. If you want to try it, make sure you use a dental dam – or a condom that's been cut open – over the anus, as you don't want to get any nasty infections. And don't let any oil – or cream, if you play this game – near the dam or condom, as it can make them break.

Ear-darting Flickering your tongue lightly in and around a man's ear can be intensely pleasurable – particularly if you team it with whispering rude things to him.

... You taste scrummy! ...

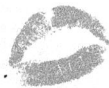

Pleasing Him

Die or dare

Men often feel uncomfortable expressing their sexual

desires, in case they seem too demanding or for fear of

being politically incorrect. This game helps men to open

up and share their raunchiest thoughts. You could well

discover a saucy side to your partner you never

realized was there …

TO PLAY

Starts by rolling a die to pick from one of the following options. Read it to your man.

1 =   Let's have sex standing up, while you support my weight and I wrap my

       legs around you.

2 =   Lie back while I lick your penis and stroke your perineum.

3 =   Stand up while I kneel in front of you and stroke your penis.

4 =   Let me rub your prostate until you reach climax.

5 =   Sit up while I kneel astride you and bite your nipples.

6 =   Let me suck and lick your testicles.

Your partner has a choice: he can either accept the option given, or go for a dare
– chosen by you – instead.

BENEFITS OF THE GAME

This game helps to build trust as, if your partner opts for a dare rather than the option offered by the die, he will be putting himself in your hands. It also helps you to extend beyond your normal sex 'comfort zone'; this will help you to avoid becoming set in your ways and getting bored.

VARIATIONS OF THE GAME

Make your own list of options for the die to choose between. Make sure you include some things that you know will push your partner's limits, so that he has to make an active decision about whether to risk a dare, rather than just settling for an easy option.

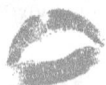

... Let's do something different ...

HOT TIP

Although men tend to be very enthusiastic about having anal sex with the woman as 'receiver', a lot tend to get nervous about having their own anus stimulated.

In fact, men are designed to get much more pleasure from anal stimulation than women, as they have the prostate – or male G-spot – a few inches inside the anus on the front wall. When rubbed in the right way, this can massively intensify a man's orgasm.

If you decide to try it, start by having a bath together. Not only does this make sure that everything is clean, which will help you both feel more comfortable, but it will also help his muscles to relax, thus making it a lot easier for you to penetrate him.

Start slowly: put lots of lube over his anus and your fingers, then run your finger round the outer rim of his anus until you feel it start to relax. As it does, slip just the tip of your finger inside. Don't force it: the anus will open up naturally as it relaxes. Make sure that any finger inserted into an anus is clean and has a short nail: ideally, use latex gloves or a condom on the toy or your fingers, to prevent infection.

As your finger slides inside, feel around for a walnut-shaped bump. Everyone is different, so you may not find it immediately. If the man says it hurts at any point, stop and slowly withdraw your finger. Or, if it's just getting a little tight, add more lube and keep your finger still until the anus relaxes again. Take your time; stroke his penis while you search and you could well end up giving him the sensation of his life.

... Put your trust in me ...

Pleasing Her

Women tend to need more foreplay than men in

order to achieve orgasm, and why not – it's fun, after all. These sexy games

will help you provide more than enough satisfaction. From oral sex to giving

that magic touch, and beyond, by playing these games you can guarantee

she'll be begging for more.

SCORE 3

Search me, sweetie!

Girls are made of sugar and spice and all things nice, or

so the old rhyme goes. This game shows how true that is,

by teaming your favourite sweet treats with your favourite woman, then

nibbling them off her. What could be a

sweeter way to spend a night?

TO PLAY

The sweet shop may seem like a strange place to go to improve your sex life, but you'd be surprised at how much fun 'penny' sweets can be for adults. Start by rolling a single die to establish which sweet you're going to play with:

1 *Sherbet Dip* The fizz makes oral sex extra-special – but careful where you put the dipper …

2 *Space Dust* Imagine the sensation of it popping over your most sensitive parts – or even sharing a kiss and feeling it pop together.

3 **Liquorice bootlace** To tie each other up, then nibble away.

4 Mars Bar With the number of stories about them, sex play with a Mars Bar has to be tried at least once.

5 A Finger of Fudge Like a Mars Bar, but smaller, leaving more options open.

6 A packet of Extra Strong Mints Makes your bits tingle as well as giving you minty fresh breath.

Once you've picked your sweet, the fun can start. Wait outside the bedroom, or close your eyes, while your partner hides the sweet somewhere on her body, tucking it into an item of clothing or even somewhere a bit racier …

   Now, roll all three dice and add them together to get a total score, and follow the instructions below. Your mission, in all cases, is to find the sweet.

3–6 Men Search for the sweet without using your hands: use your lips, tongue, elbows and even feet to search every inch of your partner's body. While it can be tempting for her just to lie back and enjoy the sensation, this game offers a great opportunity for communication. So, if you touch your woman in a way she particularly likes, she should tell you. That way, it can be incorporated into your sex play on a regular basis.

7–12 Women Use chocolate body paint or honey drizzled over your body to lead your partner to where you've hidden the sweet. But he has to lick every bit of it off before he's allowed his reward.

13–18 Men Blindfold your partner and then breathe all over her body. She then lets you know how near you are to the sweet by saying 'warmer' or 'colder' as you move around. Every time you get 'warmer', you can get more intimate: start using your tongue and lips to search, or trail your fingers softly over her body, The blindfold will heighten the sensation for her.

BENEFITS OF THE GAME

Your partner gets teased all over while you get to learn about her erogenous zones.

VARIATIONS OF THE GAME

Skip the first step and use sweets you already have in the house, but bear in mind that chocolates will get you particularly sticky! Go for a boiled sweet instead if you're really concerned about the sheets, but come on – good sex is about getting sticky together …

… Mmmm – a tasty treat …

HOT TIP

After you've got sticky together, what could be better than a sensual shower? Buy some sensually scented shower gel: sandalwood and ylang ylang are both great for boosting the libido – as if it will need it, after all that nibbling.

Soap each other down and get dirty while you're getting clean. A scalp massage is an erotic treat, so wash your partner's hair and let the pads of your fingers caress her scalp. Then let your fingers trail over her neck and back, maybe massaging her shoulders en route. As you move further down, make sure that you cover every inch of her body: after all, you don't want there to be a single drop of chocolate sauce left anywhere …

Dry each other with warm, fluffy towels, then go and get changed in private. Give your partner a final surprise by heading for the bedroom first, lighting some candles, putting on some soft music and getting out the massage oil, to finish off your massage in style. Who knows where it will lead …

… Let's get into a lather …

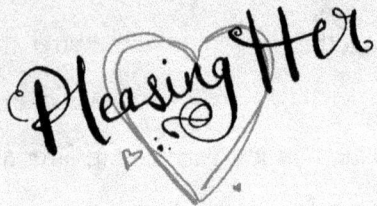

Pleasing Her

SCORE 4

Stroke me

Women tend to need more foreplay than men to get their motor running. The skin is the largest erogenous zone in the body, but many couples ignore sensual stroking, instead focusing on more direct stimulation. This game helps you to appreciate every inch of your partner's body – and will help her to reach new heights.

TO PLAY

Start by each making a numbered list of six of your favourite sexual activities. They should all be things that you could theoretically do tonight, so don't include anything that requires props or situations that you won't be able to accommodate, and stick to foreplay techniques or sexual positions.

Your partner then undresses, and is blindfolded before lying down on the bed. If she isn't comfortable about being blindfolded, ask her to lie on her front and close her eyes instead. Either way, make sure that the heating is on – you don't want her to get cold, and she's going to be there for a while.

Now, collect six different items from around the house: feather duster, clean tea towel, ice cube, paintbrush, suede cushion, cuddly toy, or whatever else you can find that has a distinctive texture or sensation about it. Don't pick any sharp items, though, for reasons that will become apparent as the game progresses.

Return to your partner and tell her that she has to guess what the item is from the way it feels alone. Every time she correctly identifies an item, she gets a point which can be redeemed against sexual favours at the end of the game, the first point winning her the first favour on her list, the second point winning the second favour, and so on. Of course, if you want to cheat you can always strip naked to distract her …

Start by trailing the item over a less sensitive part of her skin – say, the thicker skin on her knees or elbows. If she doesn't guess, progress to the back of her hand, her inner thighs and finally – gently – her genitals, If she still can't guess the item then you win a point, to be redeemed for a sexual favour on your list.

BENEFITS OF THE GAME

Your partner will have to pay far more attention than usual to her body: the blindfold will heighten her other senses to help with this.

And, depending on how sensually you trail the items over her, this game can also double as foreplay …

VARIATIONS OF THE GAME

Rather than using items from around the house, use different parts of your body – your hair, teeth, nails, penis, testicles and feet, say. She has to guess which part of your body you are using to caress her (it shouldn't be too difficult!).

If you want to make the game harder for her, you can set a time limit in which she has to identify the item (or part of the body).

HOT TIP

Generally speaking, men prefer firmer caresses to women and, as most people treat a partner as they'd like to be treated, tend to stroke women somewhat harder than is ideal.

A gentle touch can be a lot more arousing. Use just your fingertips, or softly run your hand over the delicate hairs of your partner's body. If you're not sure how much pressure to use, let your partner put her hand on yours and drag your hand over her body the way she'd most like to be stroked. You'll probably find she directs you to her ultimate erogenous zones too, so you learn twice as much.

Kissing a woman all over is another sensual treat, which will have her writhing in pleasure. Don't just use your lips: flicker your tongue over her skin, or carefully and delicately nibble her.

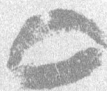

... What a stroke of genius ...

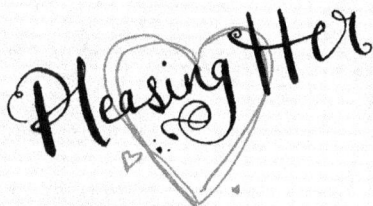

Pleasing Her

SCORE 5

Dice tease

Remember those days of teenage fumblings, when you were desperate to take things further but couldn't? This game helps bring back those memories: it's one step forwards, two steps back as you remove your partner's clothes agonizingly slowly, paying attention to every inch you reveal, of course.

TO PLAY

Write a numbered list, with each number corresponding to an item of clothing that your partner is wearing. For example, something like:

1 = skirt 3 = knickers 5 = top

2 = bra   4 = tights   6 = shoes

If she has less than six items on, repeat an item of clothing more than once on the list.

Now ask your partner to roll the die. You have to remove the item of clothing that corresponds to her die roll – but without using your hands. You can use your lips, teeth (careful about taking her underwear off with them!), elbows, feet or any other part of your body that you'd care to try. If it's an item of clothing underneath another item of clothing, you'll have to remove anything that's in the way first. If you fail to remove the designated item of clothing in an agreed amount of time – say, 10 minutes – you have to pay a sexual forfeit.

BENEFITS OF THE GAME

By taking your time removing your partner's clothes you'll get to study her body a lot more closely than usual. She may well find it a turn-on having you remove her underwear with your lips. Or you could end up laughing together, which is never a bad thing for building a bond between you.

VARIATIONS OF THE GAME

If you want to be really strict – and you totally trust each other – then the woman can tie the man's hands. Or you could take it in turns to roll the die and remove an item of each other's clothing, if she wants to get you naked, too …

HOT TIP

Once your partner has stripped off, take inspiration from ancient texts and pay homage to her body. Eastern sex texts would often include entire chapters on *Yoni* (vaginal) worship. To prove his worth, a man would have to get down on his knees and pay homage to his partner's most intimate parts, showing her his utmost devotion. According to the *Yoni Tantra* text (a Bengalese scripture from around the eleventh century):

'He should place her on his left, and should worship her hair-adorned Yoni. At the edges of the Yoni, the devotee should place sandalwood and beautiful blossoms. After smearing sandalwood on her forehead, giving her wine and drawing a half-moon using vermilion, the devotee should caress her breasts.'

But while the ancient rituals are all very well, you may find it a bit laughable to plait your partner's pubic hair with petals. Instead, focus on her body in a more up-to-date way.

Run your partner a bath, then lather up her pubic hair with her favourite shampoo. Rinse it off and then condition her, to make her hair silky smooth – and to pamper her beyond measure. Once she gets out of the bath, comb through her pubic hair to get rid of any loose hairs that could get stuck in your mouth during oral sex. Then rub some Sandalwood scented oil through her pubes for a touch of Eastern magic.

What you do next is entirely up to you: go for a genital massage (after washing your hands to remove any trace of oils, as these can irritate her sensitive skin and cause condoms to break). Or languorously lick her entire Yoni, paying particular attention to her clitoris. It's a sensual way to show how much you love your partner.

... Let me help you with your clothes ...

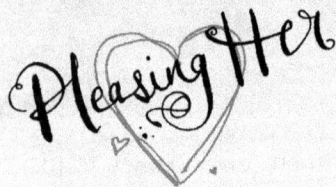

Pleasing Her

My favourite things

Women often feel uncomfortable expressing their sexual desires, in case it seems like they're being too demanding, or for fear of being seen as a tart. This game helps women to open up and share their raunchiest thoughts. Then you get to decide whether to make them come true ...

TO PLAY

Your partner starts by rolling a die to choose from the following options:

1 = cunnilingus technique

2 = masturbation technique

3 = sexual position

4 = sexy outfit for partner to wear

5 = fantasy

6 = body part to be stimulated, excluding genitals

She then writes down her favourite thing in the category selected: say, being licked slowly from the labia to the tip of her clitoris, or making love with the man on top.

You then have to guess what she has chosen – either by asking questions or by demonstrating what you think her answer will be, while your partner says 'hotter' or 'colder' depending on how close you're getting to picking the option that she's written down.

She should be as specific as possible when writing down her options: the more detail she goes into, the longer the game will take and the more fun you'll both have. It also means that you'll get to learn more about exactly what it is that really turns your woman on.

BENEFITS OF THE GAME

If your partner goes into detail about the things that she most enjoys in the bedroom, you will learn how to please her best when you're getting intimate. And by playing a game rather than simply having a conversation, it's less confrontational and much easier for both of you.

HOT TIP

All women like being praised. One sexy way to do this is by emulating Leonardo diCaprio in Titanic, and drawing a picture of your lover while you tell her how gorgeous she is. Get her to recline on a couch, wearing her favourite lingerie – or nothing at all – then get out a sketchbook (or easel if you're feeling really ambitious!) and begin to create an artistic impression of her. Don't worry about your technical skills: the important thing here is the compliments that you pay your partner in the process. (You could always skip the sketching if you prefer – just don't skip the compliments!)

Don't just go for the obvious: most women are aware of at least one of their body parts that men tend to like. For some, it's their breasts, for others their legs. You certainly shouldn't ignore your partner's favourite feature, but she'll feel even more cherished if you tell her that you love the way that her hair curls into the nape of her neck, adore the freckle on her lower back or find the way that she crinkles her nose when she laughs adorable. Think of compliments that she's never heard before: you can guarantee that she'll remember them – and you'll probably win brownie points with her friends too, because she'll undoubtedly tell them all about your romantic gesture.

And don't be coy about praising her genitals, either. Many women feel uncomfortable about their most intimate parts, so telling her that you think she has beautiful labia or incredible pubic hair will help her to feel more sexually confident; and let's face it, you're in a privileged position to be able to give her a compliment like that.

... You've made a real impression on me ...

Pleasing Her

You forgot this!

Remember the game where you place items on a tray, ask someone to memorize them then remove one and see if they can remember what you've removed? This game adds a sexy twist – and you can guarantee that your partner's memory will improve when she sees what you do with the items …

TO PLAY

Start by filling a tray with at least ten sexy items. They don't all have to be obviously designed for sex: you could include things like a jar of honey for drizzling over your partner's genitals; or a silk scarf to run sensually over her body. Other items could include a sex toy, a pair of handcuffs or a tie for bondage fun, a feather, a bottle of lubricant, a condom, an erotic book or sexy video – basically anything that you can use in your sex play.

Now, give your partner a minute to memorize all of the items on the tray. Ask her to turn away or close her eyes at the end of the minute, then remove one of the items and place it out of view. She now has to guess which item is missing. If she guesses correctly, she wins a sexual favour of her choice. But if she gets it wrong, things get really interesting …

Put the missing item back on the tray, and then give a demonstration of exactly how each item can be used in your sex play: for example, tie your partner down and tease her clitoris while she's unable to wriggle away, massage her labia using the lube, or read her a passage from the erotic book. Work your way through all ten items, giving her only a brief taster of the joy that they can give her. Once you've demonstrated all ten items, and she's desperate with anticipation, tell her to close her eyes again and remove one of the items. After you've shown her exactly what you can do with each item, you can guarantee she'll find it a lot easier to remember. And she'll be more than anxious to win her sexual favour …

BENEFITS OF THE GAME

Not only do you get to experiment with lots of fun accessories but this game will also help your partner form kinky mental associations with all the items on the tray. She'll smile every time she sees the jar of honey in the cupboard!

VARIATIONS OF THE GAME

To make the game easier or harder, vary the number of items that you use, or the amount of time you give your partner to memorize them. Or, write down different sex acts on a piece of paper and get her to memorize those instead – and, if necessary, demonstrate them all. You could make her pay you a sexual forfeit if she can't guess the item, before you go on to prompt her memory.

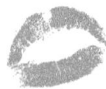

... You won't forget this in a hurry! ...

HOT TIP

Keep the romance in your relationship by making a memory-prompt book. For example, if you go on holiday and have a particularly steamy session on the beach, buy a postcard of that beach and stick it into the book, writing a brief description of what happened underneath it.

If you buy your partner some lingerie that she particularly loves, take a picture of her in it and stick that in the book. Write down the dates of your birthdays and anniversaries, and note down any particularly sexy treats that you've given your partner on those days,

By keeping a record of the good sex that you have, you've got something to refer back to if things start to slip. And it also acts as a fun form of foreplay: looking through the book together will remind you of all your hottest nights and help you get aroused remembering the good times.

... Fancy a good read? ...

Pleasing Her

SCORE 8

Win, lose or strip

It's a classic card game, but this time with a twist. The woman
has to remove her clothes in the usual way, while the man – rather than just
stripping off – has to pay a forfeit as well, every time he loses a hand. This is
one game that can get really steamy …

TO PLAY

Use a standard pack of playing cards and deal each person two cards. Add up your score – an ace can equate to 1 or 11 and picture cards are worth 10. The aim of the game is to score 21. Take it in turns to decide whether to add another card (twist) or stay with the cards you have (stick). Whoever scores closest to 21, without going over it, wins the hand.

If the woman loses the hand, she has to remove an item of clothing. If the man loses the hand, he also has to remove an item of clothing – and pay a sexual forfeit of the woman's choice. All forfeits should last no longer than 2 minutes – set an alarm to make sure that you stick to the time allocation, as it prolongs the teasing.

The game continues until you've used all the cards in the pack – or until neither of you can resist taking things a little further …

BENEFITS OF THE GAME

This game makes foreplay last for ages – always a good thing if you want to increase the chance of a woman having an orgasm. The game will also show you exactly what a woman wants – and how mean she is when it comes to choosing forfeits!

VARIATIONS OF THE GAME

You can add a stripping and forfeit element to any game of cards. Pick your favourite game to play. Or, if cards aren't your thing (or you don't have a deck to hand), try it with other quick games, like Noughts and Crosses.

... You'll always score with me ...

HOT TIP

As this game has a gambling theme, why not take things further and indulge in the classic fantasy of making love on a bed covered in money? It takes a little preparation (unless you're loaded) but the decadent feeling is worth it …

First, you'll need to go out to buy some fake money. You could make your own, but do be aware that it's illegal to photocopy currency in the UK, so unless you want to come up with your own bank-note design it's much easier to use fake stuff. Either that, or go to the bank and exchange some money for a foreign currency that has a good exchange rate – a million will still feel like a lot of money, even if it's worth very little!

Play up to the fantasy by getting dressed up in your foxiest clothes: the man can wear a suit while the woman wears a sexy dress and all her glitziest jewellery. It's easy enough to pretend that diamanté is diamonds in the heat of the moment.

Have a bottle of champagne or sparkling wine chilling in an ice bucket next to the bed, and add to the decadence with a box of Belgian chocolates, smoked salmon or even caviar.

The exact nature of the fantasy is up to you. Maybe you are dissolute and debauched millionaires living out your base desires. Or perhaps you're villains on the run after a heist, taking advantage of the moment before the police turn up to arrest you. Or maybe it's a scenario in which one of you has paid the other a million pounds for a night of passion.

Whichever fantasy you pick, make sure you get into character: imagination is there to be used, and you may well find that it jolts you out of your usual sexual habits. And who knows, you may even discover whether it's true that you get what you pay for ...

... What would you do for a million? ...

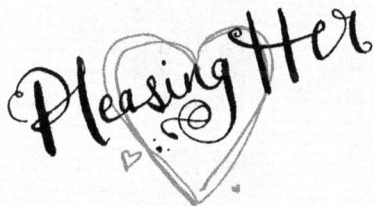

Pleasing Her

Tongue twister

Oral sex is incredibly popular with many women, but all too often men just rely on one technique. This game will teach you new ways to pleasure a woman with your lips and tongue and, in doing so, introduce variety to your lovemaking experience. Just make sure you pay attention to the techniques she really loves …

TO PLAY

First, roll a die to pick from one of the following techniques:

1 = under the tongue. Use the soft underside of your lips to rub the woman's clitoris. This gives a softer sensation than using your tongue. You may find it easiest if you use your fingers to hold back the woman's clitoral hood to expose her sensitive clitoral tip. Some women find this too sensitive, though, so go gently.

2 = sucking. Try gently sucking the clitoris between your lips, increasing the suction as she gets more aroused. Don't suck too hard, though, as it can be painful. Changing from intense sucking to barely perceptible sucking can be a sensual tease.

3 = French kissing. If you roll a 3, try 'French kissing' her vagina; dart your tongue in and out. Adding a few appreciative comments about how wonderful your partner tastes will add to the experience for her, too.

4 = labia lover. The inner labia are rooted at the clitoral hood, and nibbling, licking or sucking on them indirectly stimulates the clitoris, and will help build a woman's arousal. Try massaging the outer labia with your fingers at the same time, to add extra thrills.

5 = penetration. Flex and curl your tongue, then insert it into her vaginal opening, and thrust it at a rhythm that works for both of you. Teaming this with fingers can deliver mind-blowing results, especially if you use a 'come-here' motion with them to stimulate her G-spot.

6 = tongue nudge. Try nudging back the clitoral hood with your tongue, with incredibly light pressure, Then use just the tip of your tongue to delicately dart over the head of her clitoris. Moistening your little finger and using the tip of it can also be pleasurable.

BENEFITS OF THE GAME

Different oral sex techniques give different sensations, so you may well discover new ways to pleasure your partner. And having various techniques to choose from means that when your tongue gets tired of one technique, you can move on to another. Needless to say, your partner will really appreciate your new-found skills, too.

VARIATIONS OF THE GAME

Buy a sex manual with more oral sex techniques and give yourself different options to choose from. The more techniques you have to choose from, the better your lovemaking is likely to be.

... Looks like I'm a bit tongue-tied ...

HOT TIP

Other ways to add to oral sex include things like:

- Softly blowing across a woman's clitoris – but never up the vagina, as this can be dangerous.
- Gently pulling her pubic hair to part her lips and give a pain/ pleasure thrill.
- Humming on the clitoris to add vibrations to the experience.
- Alternating thrusting your tongue with sucking the clitoris and licking her labia – varying techniques will stop your tongue getting too tired.

Don't just stick to the same position, either. Going in from the top allows you to stimulate the whole of the clitoris rather than just the tip, which may be good if a woman is sensitive. Or go from behind to team cunnilingus with anal teasing. No matter what position you go for, one thing is essential: shave first – otherwise she'll feel like you're rubbing sandpaper over her most sensitive parts.

Pleasing Her

Do or dare

When it comes to getting wild, women can sometimes feel uncomfortable about their desires: after all, a lot of women are still brought up to believe 'good girls' don't like sex. This game helps you tap into a woman's wilder desires – and helps her learn where her own limits are.

TO PLAY

Start by rolling a die to pick from one of the following options to read to your partner.

1 =   Let's have anal sex.

2 =   Lie back while I push back your clitoral hood and lick the tip of your clitoris.

3 =   Stand up while I kneel down in front of you and perform oral sex.

4 =   Let me rub your G-spot until you reach climax.

5 =   Sit up while I kneel astride you and bite your nipples.

6 =   Let me suck and lick your feet.

Once the die has chosen one of the options, your partner has a choice: she can either accept the option given, or go for a dare – chosen by you – instead.

BENEFITS OF THE GAME

This game helps build trust, as your partner will be putting herself completely in your hands if she dislikes one of the options offered by the die and decides to opt for a dare instead. It also helps you extend outside your normal 'comfort zone' of sex, which will help you avoid getting too set in your ways and ending up bored.

VARIATIONS OF THE GAME

Come up with your own list of options for the die to choose between. Make sure that you include some things that you know will push your partner's limits, so that she will have to make an active decision about whether to risk a dare, rather than just settling for an easy option.

HOT TIP

Only ten per cent of couples practise anal sex, so don't feel that it's something you're obliged to do. However, if the woman is willing to try it, a few things can make it easier for the man and more comfortable for the woman.

Start by having a bath together, so that you're both clean and relaxed. Then devote some time to anal foreplay. Lube is an essential for anal play – silicone-based ones are best, as they are the most slippery.

Start by caressing the outside of the woman's anus and, as she relaxes, you'll feel it start to open and let your finger in. Go slowly, letting her anus get used to the feeling of your finger before you push it forward. If it hurts her at any point, stop. If it's just tight, add more lube and keep your finger still until her anus relaxes again.

Once she's comfortably taking your finger, try adding another one – again, going slowly and using lots of lube. The more she's got used to beforehand, the easier it will be for her to take your penis.

If and when she feels ready, put on a condom (the anus has much thinner skin than the vagina and can get damaged more easily, so safer sex is even more important), and press the head of the penis against the anus. Again, wait for it to welcome your penis in. The first inch or so is the hardest, but rushing things will make it impossible as she'll tighten up. Keep pushing slowly forward if your partner's comfortable with it, and then thrust away – but more gently than normal. Voilà! You're having anal sex.

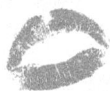

... *Shall we give it a try?* ...

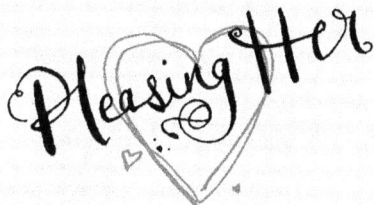

Pleasing Her

SCORE 11

Change the pace

Different strokes for different folks, or so the old saying goes. But it's surprising how many people don't bother to vary the rhythm when they're performing sex acts, instead using the same speed with every partner. This game helps you find out how fast or slow your partner really wants to go.

TO PLAY

Pick six songs that you like and that you have in the house. Make sure that they are each of a different tempo: say, a romantic song, a fast dance number, a classical piece, or whatever else you are into.

Get the CDs out, and write down each of the song titles, numbering them from 1 to 6. Now, roll a die to pick a song. Then roll again to decide which sex act:

1–2 = manual stimulation

3–4 = oral sex

5–6 = penetrative sex

You have to perform the sex act indicated in time to the piece of music. Remember – this game has the woman's pleasure in mind, so it's the man who takes control: the woman simply lies back and enjoys herself. If a certain song isn't working, roll the die again and select another song.

BENEFITS OF THE GAME

By varying the rhythm with which you perform sex acts, you change the sensation: fast sex is often deeper, too, whereas slow sex can be more sensual. A romantic tune will give you time to deliver lingering oral sex, while a dance number may be better suited to deeper thrusting. Most people tend to use a consistent rhythm when they make love, so miss out on the infinite pleasures afforded by ringing the changes.

VARIATIONS OF THE GAME

Put the radio or music television on instead, and vary the pace of your lovemaking to fit with each new song that comes on. Or, if you don't have a stereo or TV in the bedroom, imagine the song going through your head – or get your partner to sing to you, if you're sure it won't ruin her concentration!

HOT TIP

Women tend to find it harder to climax than men, and changing rhythm all the time can be less than helpful. When you're performing a sex act, the golden rule is: if it seems to be working, don't change what you're doing! Many an orgasm has been lost by a man changing rhythm for variety just as the woman's approaching the point of no return.

Communicating throughout sex is the best solution to this, though the woman should be the one saying whether she wants the man to speed up or slow down when he's performing oral sex (if the man stops to ask 'Is this OK?' midway through, it can be counter-productive). But at all other times, if you're unsure whether what you're doing is hitting the spot, ask. If you know each other well enough to have sex, you know each other well enough to talk about it.

... Let's get into the rhythm ...

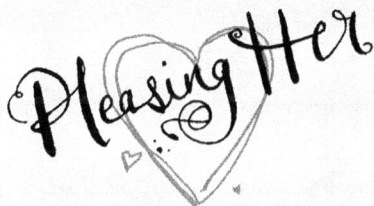

Pleasing Her

SCORE 12

Sweet sensations

Food can be a sensual addition to sex. Through smothering your woman in your favourite sweet treats and eating them off her naked body, you'll learn where she most likes to be licked; and, in the meantime, you get to enjoy your just desserts …

TO PLAY

This game takes a bit of planning but it's worth it. Start by going shopping for all your favourite sweet treats: ice-cream, whipped cream, mousse, fresh fruit, chocolate sauce and anything else that takes your fancy.

Next, put a plastic sheet or a cut-open bin bag on the floor. Get your partner to lie down on it and create the dessert of your dreams on her naked body. Treat this as foreplay: drizzle chocolate sauce slowly over her thighs, and pour whipped cream over her breasts while you caress her nipples, or put chocolate buttons, strawberries or cherries on her clitoris, rolling them around as you do so to stimulate her. Try peeling a grape, softly pressing back her clitoral hood and running the grape over her exposed clitoris.

Once you've got your partner suitably smothered in your favourite treats, lick, suck and nibble them off. The chances are you'll both get pretty messy –

but that's half the fun of the game. And if you get too sticky, she can always clean you off with her tongue.

BENEFITS OF THE GAME

She gets lots of foreplay while you get to enjoy your favourite dessert! And there's nothing to stop you from feeding her food while you decorate her – from your lips as you nibble it off.

VARIATIONS OF THE GAME

Get your partner to lie in the bath rather than on a plastic sheet while you 'decorate' her – then get in there and start eating, before filling the bath up to clean each other off.

And, if you don't have a sweet tooth, use savoury food like cheese spread from a tube, olives and cucumber instead. Avoid anything spicy, though, because it can sting and cause irritation.

HOT TIP

Combining a mixture of warm and cold foods can make this game even sexier (and the dessert even tastier!). Obviously, you don't want to use anything that's hot enough to burn, but putting a spoonful of ice-cream over a woman's clitoris then sucking it off, before spooning over some warm fudge sauce, can be deliciously decadent.

Think of the texture of the foods that you're using, too: combine slippery sauces to trickle over her labia with moist fruit to rub over her clitoris, and maybe even add a rougher touch with a wafer to scrape sauce off her nipples. Put chocolate somewhere on her body where it will melt from her body heat and let it get sticky before you lick it from her.

NB It should go without saying, but do make sure your partner doesn't have any allergies before you play this game; the last thing you want to do is trigger an allergic reaction.

... I always save room for dessert ...

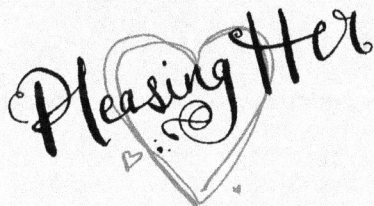

Pleasing Her

SCORE 13

Touch me this way

Think you know exactly how your partner wants to be touched?

Are you prepared to put it to the test? This game helps you

see exactly how well you know your partner. And she gets

to enjoy the erotic sensation of a paintbrush tickling

her most sensitive parts …

TO PLAY

For this game, surprisingly enough, you'll need body paints. You can get paint specially designed for body painting or just use children's face-painting crayons. The former is preferable as they're applied with a brush, which is much more sensual than a crayon.

Your partner starts by drawing a picture of her body, without you seeing it. She then labels each body part with the act that she most likes having performed on it: she could write 'lick' next to her neck, say, or 'scratch' on her thighs.

Once she's finished labelling her picture, she puts it into an envelope and strips naked. Make sure that the room is warm, as she'll be naked for a while and you don't want her getting goose bumps. You then begin to paint on her body – but there's a twist. Rather than just drawing pictures on her, paint words speci-fying what you think she most likes having done to that body part: for example, you could paint the word 'nibble' on her thighs, or 'suck' over her clitoris.

Once you have completed your masterpiece, your partner opens the envelope and compares your guesses with her answers. You get a point for every answer you get right, to be redeemed against sexual favours.

BENEFITS OF THE GAME

Not only does this game help you learn what your partner most wants done to her body, but the sensation of the brush or paints will also give her a sensual thrill in the process.

VARIATIONS OF THE GAME

If you don't have any body paints, you can just use lipstick or eyeliner to paint your partner's body.

... Let me paint your desires ...

HOT TIP

This game can be added to if the woman shaves off her pubic hair: that way the man can paint over every inch of her body. A few tips will make this a lot easier and make itchy grow-back less likely.

Make sure you use a new razor, shaving foam or oil and lots of clean water. Be careful not to get any foam or oil in the vagina, as it will cause irritation. Use lukewarm rather than hot water, as it dries out skin less, which will help prevent irritation. If the razor starts to dull, use a new one, After shaving, splash the pubic area thoroughly with cold water to remove all traces of foam and tighten up the pores. A mild astringent (not alcohol-based, as it will sting) may also help.

Next, dry yourself off with a soft towel and use lots of gentle moisturizer. Baby lotion (not oil – that will block the pores) is ideal. Whatever you use, make sure it's designed for sensitive skin, as you can't get a lot more sensitive than the skin on your pubic mound. Aftercare is important. Keep moisturizing until the hair's long enough not to cause irritation (around 3–4 days). It will also help if you don't wear any knickers for a few days, and avoid wearing jeans or tights.

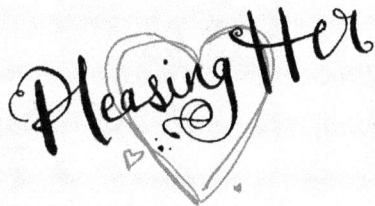

Pleasing Her

SCORE 14

Slow hand

There are numerous different ways to pleasure a woman

using your hands, but lots of men rely solely on thrusting a finger in and out.

This game helps you explore a variety of techniques – and find out which one

gets your partner to melt the most.

TO PLAY

Start by rolling a die to choose from one of the following techniques to perform on your partner:

1 = loving the pearl. You may choose to start with this as your preferred technique. *Loving the pearl* works more effectively when your partner is getting really aroused. Rest your thumb and index finger on either side of her clitoris and rub it back and forth. Follow her body movements to set the pace.

2 = treat her like a man. Try masturbating the clitoris as if it was a miniature penis. Not all women have a large enough clitoris for this to be possible; if your partner is one of them, simply put your fingers on either side of her clitoris and rub or squeeze it.

3 = drumming. Try drumming your fingers against your partner's pubic mound and clitoris. This will send vibrations though her most sensitive parts.

4 = twirling. Twirl her labia between your fingers as if you were twirling a piece of string.

5 = the stir. This is a sensual technique that many women enjoy. Using your index and middle fingers together, insert them into her vagina, then 'stir' them around to tease her vaginal walls. You may want to combine this with G-spot stimulation to add to her pleasure.

6 = stroking. Try softly stroking your partner's clitoris, focusing on the clitoral hood to start with, until she starts to get aroused. Some women don't like direct clitoral stimulation until just before they climax, and others don't like the tip being touched at all as it can be too sensitive. Work around the base of the clitoris and her inner lips if this is the case. Even if she likes direct clitoral stimulation, she'll appreciate you taking a gradual approach to reach it.

BENEFITS OF THE GAME

Every woman is different, so by trying some new techniques you could discover a turn-on that you – and your partner – never realized was there before. And variety is the spice of life, after all.

VARIATIONS OF THE GAME

Buy a sex manual and make alternative numbered lists of different clitoral and vaginal stimulation techniques to choose from.

... Fancy trying something new? ...

HOT TIP

Using your fingers to stimulate a woman is rarely about penetration alone. Indeed, you shouldn't penetrate her vagina with your fingers until she's lubricated, as it can be painful. It can be easier for a woman to climax through manual stimulation than through pene-trative sex, as your fingers can be far more precise than your penis, hitting her most sensitive zones. You can caress her G-spot, A-zone and clitoris.

The clitoris has the sole function of giving a woman sexual pleasure – and it's far bigger than you might think. It's wishbone- shaped, with three-quarters of it hidden from view. But, while the clitoris is important, it's not the be-all and end-all. The labia and entire pubic area are very responsive too. Spend time stroking your partner's pubic mound or running your fingers over her labia. You can rest assured that she'll appreciate your efforts.

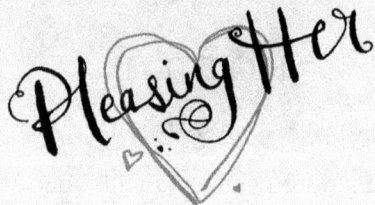

Pleasing Her

SCORE 15

Show and tell

Most men find the idea of a woman pleasuring herself in

front of them immensely arousing, but it's also a great way

for them to learn. In this game, the woman shows the man what to do, then

awards him points for how quickly he learns

– to be redeemed against sexual favours, of course …

TO PLAY

Start by rolling a die to choose from one of the following options:

1–2 = fingers

3–4 = sex toy

5–6 = some other method

Your partner then picks the way in which she masturbates in front of you, based on the roll of the die. If she only ever reaches orgasm in one particular way – say, with her fingers – then this stage can be skipped.

You then prepare a comfortable area in which your woman can recline – this is a game for her, after all – maybe scattering some cushions on the floor and giving her a throw to wrap around herself should she get cold. Light some candles and dim the lights to create an air of romance; this can also help less confident women to feel more comfortable about what they are doing.

Your partner then lies back and masturbates in the manner chosen by the die. You should sit near enough to see the action close-up, and to allow her to reach for your hand to touch herself.

Once she is getting aroused, she should place your hand where she would most like it to be. If she wants you to take over pleasuring her genitals, you can – but she has to keep her hand on top of yours to control the speed, pressure and the way in which you touch her. Every time you get a stroke right, she can give you a point – to be redeemed against sexual favours.

BENEFITS OF THE GAME

By seeing how your partner masturbates, you will learn exactly how she wants to be touched. This game also builds intimacy, as masturbation is usually a private thing.

VARIATIONS OF THE GAME

Both partners can masturbate and watch the way that the other person pleasures themselves, before moving on to help each other out. Or, the woman can masturbate in front of a mirror, so that both partners can see what's going on.

... Do it this way, on reflection ...

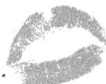

HOT TIP

There are numerous masturbation techniques a woman can use and, even if you've been masturbating for years, there may be some variations that will make things even better. Try some of these to see if there's a new way to pleasure yourself you've never experienced before:

- Stroking the hood of the clitoris to stimulate the clitoris underneath it.
- Gently tugging your pubes upwards to move your clitoral hood up and down over your clitoris.
- Putting one finger on either side of your clitoris and pleasuring it as if it's a miniature penis.
- Moving your finger rapidly from side to side over your clitoris.
- Circling your finger around the tip of your clitoris.
- Pushing the clitoral hood gently back and stroking the tip of your clitoris.
- Stroking around your labia majora (outer lips) and/or labia minora (inner lips), both of which are densely packed with nerve endings.

- Gently pinching your labia majora and/or clitoris.

- Rubbing your labia majora together.

- Tapping your clitoris with one finger.

- Gently slapping your pubic mound and/or labia.

- Stretching open your labia majora with one hand and stroking your clitoris and/or labia minora with the other hand.

If you like penetration, try one of these finger-penetration variations:

- Sliding one or more fingers in and out slowly.

- Alternating two fingers piston-style.

- Slipping a finger or more inside you and flexing your pelvic floor muscles around it.

- Moving one or more fingers inside yourself in a circular motion.

- Holding your wrist with one hand and using it to push a finger or fingers of the other hand inside yourself.

- Putting just the tip of your finger inside yourself and moving it rapidly in and out.

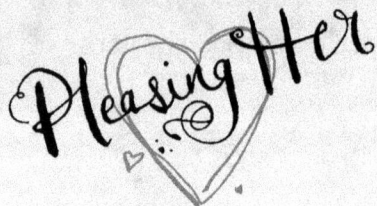

Pleasing Her

Hands-free

It can be easy to fall into the same patterns of sexual behaviour. This game

helps you use your imagination and learn new ways to pleasure your partner.

And the tricks you learn come in useful for when your tongue or

fingers get too tired, too ...

TO PLAY

Start by rolling a die to select one of the following options:

1 = nose 3 = thigh 5 = testicles

2 = feet 4 = penis 6 = wrist

Now, stimulate your woman using that part of your body alone, until she reaches climax. If the option you've chosen just isn't doing the trick, or if you get too tired using one body part, roll the die again to choose another one. Get creative: for example, if you roll a 3, maybe get the woman to straddle your thigh and grind against it. If you roll a 4, try using the penis to stimulate the nipples and neck, as well as the vagina.

Bear in mind that if you roll a 4 or a 5, you should make sure that you wear a condom unless you've both been tested for STIs and are protected against pregnancy; the head of the penis has over 3 million sperm on it, so it's not worth taking any risks. And if you roll a 2, check that the skin on your feet isn't too rough before you begin, as you don't want to snag your partner's most delicate skin.

BENEFITS OF THE GAME

By learning how to stimulate your partner with every inch of your body, you'll add variety to your lovemaking. Different body parts will give very different sensations, too.

VARIATIONS OF THE GAME

Make your own list of different body parts with which to stimulate your partner: your hair, elbow or anything else you care to come up with.

... I want you to feel a part of me ...

HOT TIP

In addition to being a fun game in its own right, this game teaches you techniques that are ideal for those times when a woman's in the mood but her partner isn't.

Rather than just lying back and getting sexually frustrated, the woman can masturbate and, as she gets more aroused, move to straddle the man's thigh. While she presses against it, he can simply relax – though there's a reasonable chance that he'll get aroused when he feels her wetness over his thigh, and things will end up progressing …

By masturbating using a part of the man's body, there's an increased feeling of closeness and intimacy which masturbating 'solo' doesn't provide. In addition, the fact that he's joining in helps to stop the man from feeling guilty for not 'performing', which is more likely to keep your sex life on track longer-term. After all, no one wants to feel that they're disappointing their partner.

Pleasing Her

SCORE 17

Don't you dare come!

The human body is a perverse thing: tell it not to do

something and that will be all that it craves. By tapping into this, you can give

your partner the climax of her life. Though obviously, that's not the aim of this

game at all …

TO PLAY

Start by rolling a die to pick from the following options:

1 = licking the clitoris   4 = licking the labia

2 = manually stimulating   5 = rubbing the pubic

the clitoris   mound

3 = manually stimulating   6 = penetrating the vagina the labia

Now, ask your partner to lie back, and administer whatever pleasure the die has dictated. But while you're doing so, look her in the eye and tell her that she's not allowed to come. As she gets nearer climax, slow your movements and reiterate your command. This isn't a game to be rushed.Take your time pleasuring her, taking her repeatedly to the edge of orgasm and then back again. If you spend enough time making her wait, then when you eventually relinquish control and tell her she can come, you may find that it happens instantly!

BENEFITS OF THE GAME

In playing this game, the man is tapping into the woman's subconscious mind. Many women feel guilty about enjoying sexual pleasure, so by banning her from having it the man is – conversely – helping her relax enough to climax. The woman can also get an extra thrill from doing something 'forbidden'.

VARIATIONS OF THE GAME

Make a list of the woman's favourite sexual techniques, and use these to roll the die against. The more effective the technique is at making her achieve climax, the crueller the game – and the more intense her eventual orgasm will be.

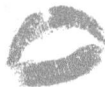

... Wait for it! ...

HOT TIP

Sex toys can be a fun addition to this game, as they deliver intense sensations, making it even harder for a woman to hold back her climax. If you've never used a sex toy before, start with something like the Jessica Rabbit: it combines penetration with clitoral stimulation, giving women a double thrill. It can also be turned round so that the clitoral stimulator teases the anus, if that's one of your partner's hot spots.

When using a toy for the first time, begin with it on the lowest setting. Sometimes the vibrations can still be too intense for a beginner; if you find that this is the case, use it through underwear or even jeans, to help tone down the sensation.

Some men are uncomfortable about their partner using a sex toy. If this is the case, maybe go with something small and non-phallic, as this can be less threatening. You can now get toys in every shape – even remote-controlled ones! Alternatively, you could experiment with a vibrating cock ring. This fits around the base of the penis and vibrates, giving dual stimulation to both partners. It also helps a man maintain his erection for longer – and it will be harder, too.

Pleasing Her

SCORE 18

Stay outside

Penetration alone isn't enough for most women to achieve climax, and yet it still forms the crux of the sex act for many couples. This game teaches you a variety of techniques for giving a woman pleasure without penetrating her at all – sure to come in useful in your future lovemaking sessions.

TO PLAY

Start by rolling a die to choose from the following options:

1 = rubbing the pubic mound with the flat of the hand

2 = squeezing the outer labia together using two fingers

3 = pushing the pubic mound up with one hand and stimulating the clitoris with the fingers of the other hand

4 = pulling the outer labia outwards while stroking the inner labia with the fingers of the other hand

5 = licking between the labia

6 = sucking the clitoris

Now, follow the directions given by the die. If your partner dislikes the technique, you should roll again to try a different option. The game continues until the woman has reached climax.

BENEFITS OF THE GAME

Women are much more likely to climax from clitoral stimulation and foreplay in general than they are from penetrative sex. By learning new ways to pleasure your partner through playing this game, you can incorporate into normal lovemaking any techniques that are particularly effective – added to which, this game is likely to result in orgasm for the woman, which is always a good thing.

VARIATIONS OF THE GAME

Pick six options that are purely based around clitoral stimulation: for example, sucking on the clitoris, licking it with the underside of the tongue, breathing on it while holding the clitoral hood back, rubbing it with one finger, rubbing it with the entire hand and squeezing it between two fingers. Or pick six labia techniques – or even anal ones, if the woman enjoys that activity.

HOT TIP

There are numerous ways to pleasure a woman manually. Try using the flat of all of your fingers to massage the labia, or pressing the heel of your hand against your partner's pubic area while she writhes against it. Letting her set the pace will help make both of your lives a lot easier.

Pressing one hand against a woman's pubic bone, with the heel of the hand resting on top of her ovaries while you stimulate her with your fingers, can help deepen her orgasm. And try rocking your hand back and forth as you do so; it will help stretch her skin and indirectly stimulate the clitoris.

Once your partner is aroused enough, she may want you to penetrate her with your fingers or with a sex toy. Start slowly, with just one finger, a joint at a time, or just the tip of the toy: contrary to popular belief, women don't necessarily just want to be filled by something big. Only add more fingers (or slide the vibrator deeper inside her) when it becomes easy and she's happy for you to continue. Every woman will have her own preference as to how many fingers she likes inside her. Ask your partner if she'd like more fingers, and keep adding them at her request!

Vary the speed and the rhythm of your fingers inside her, and combine this with movements over her clitoris and playing with her nipples with your fingers or tongue. And don't just thrust in and out. Experiment with different motions, crossing and uncrossing two fingers inside your partner, or alternating them 'piston-style'. A twist of the wrist can also add a delicious thrill.

... You're bound to find this stimulating ...

Hot Positions

There are hundreds of different sexual positions to try, but

very few couples experiment with them. These games are designed to get you

thinking creatively about the various

ways in which you can make love – and to help you

find new positions you both adore.

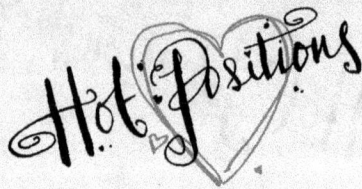

Hot Positions

SCORE 3

Statues

Everyone has their own favourite position, but does your lover know what
yours is? In this game, you give them a hint – and if they get it right? Well,
their reward is to get to continue where the game leaves off, of course. It's a
win–win scenario.

TO PLAY

Remember the old game 'Statues', in which you have to hold a position for as long as possible? Well, this version has a naughty edge to it. The woman starts by writing down the name of one of her favourite sex positions, but keeping it hidden from her partner. She then gets into the position that she would be in when trying that sex position.

The man then has to work out which sex position she's referring to, and assume his place in the position. If he gets it right, you can take the game from there and move into actually having sex in that position. If not, you have two choices: he either has to keep changing his position until he's correctly guessed which sex position the woman is referring to, or you can have sex from the position that he's assumed. You can't lose!

The next time you play, it's the man's turn to choose his favourite position and the woman's turn to guess.

BENEFITS OF THE GAME

You can find out how well you know your partner and learn what each other's favourite positions are. And you never know – you may discover some new sex positions while you're guessing.

VARIATIONS OF THE GAME

If you find that this game can only be played once or twice before you've exhausted all your favourite sexual positions, you should experiment some more (see Hot Tip). Admittedly, some adventurous positions require a bit more concentration than the plain old missionary, but they really are worth the effort. Just be careful if you've got any back injuries: if it hurts, stop.

HOT TIP

Try some of these positions to add spice to your sex life.

The Chain If you're into G-spot stimulation, join the chain gang! In this position, the woman lies on her back with her legs spread widely apart, much as she would in the missionary position. The man lies on top of her facing her feet, then lowers himself so that his feet are on either side of her shoulders and his legs are over her hips.

The woman wraps her legs around the man's back as he thrusts into her backwards. The woman can pull on his hips to deepen penetration. However, be careful. The unusual angle isn't for everyone, and you don't want to break him!

The Crane For limber lovers, The Crane is a great position. The woman stands facing her partner, who should have his legs a few feet apart to assist his balance (a wall can also come in handy). Rest your arms on his shoulders, while he supports your lower back with his hands.

Now, the tricky bit! Raise one leg up to rest on his shoulder. Once your partner is inside you, raise your leg as high as possible in a vertical split. The higher you can move your calf up his shoulder, the deeper the penetration.

The Wheelbarrow Want a real rush of lust? Get into The Wheelbarrow. Start in doggie style. The man then lifts the woman's legs, 'wheelbarrow race' style, and penetrates her. Bear in mind that the blood will rush to the woman's head, so be careful and stop if your head spins too much; fainting during sex doesn't add any thrill to the proceedings.

... Can you guess how I like it? ...

Hot Positions

Furniture fun

Sex doesn't always have to take place in bed: adding a

twist by using different items of furniture can help you reach the parts that

bed-sex alone doesn't. Whether it's making

love on the washing machine during the spin cycle, having

sex over the kitchen table or getting it on on the sofa,

you're sure to have fun experimenting.

TO PLAY

First roll a die to choose from one of the following options:

1 = sofa	4 = kitchen worksurface
2 = washing machine	5 = chair
3 = table	6 = shower

Now, between you, work out the different sex positions that are available to you using each of the items of furniture. For example, you could bend over the arm of the sofa, or the woman could sit on it while the man kneels between her legs. You could sit on the washing machine or bend over it, lean over the kitchen table or lie on it with your legs over the edge, and sit on the kitchen surface or lie on it with your legs raised …

Get creative rather than just going for the obvious. Then, try it out! If your first position doesn't hit the spot, move on to another one from your list. And if it's still not doing the trick, roll the die again to choose a different item of furniture.

BENEFITS OF THE GAME

By using furniture, you're injecting variety into your lovemaking, which will help keep things fresh. In addition, you'll find that different items of furniture make different positions easier: for example, standing doggie-style sex over the edge of the sofa can make it easier to get deep penetration, as the woman has some-thing to grip onto.

VARIATIONS OF THE GAME

Make a list of all the items of furniture in your house, and roll the die against that list. Or get really complex and make a list of six positions for each item of furniture in your house and then work your way through the whole lot. Just make sure you don't stain anything permanently!

HOT TIP

You can now get furniture that's specifically designed to enhance sex. 'Loving Angles' sex furniture (www.loving-angles.com) is a collection of differently shaped firm foam pieces that look innocent enough to be used as normal furniture but have a kinky secret. The large wedges can be placed underneath the hips to raise them up and help make penetration deeper, while the cube rocks from side to side, helping a man's thrusting action. Their smaller wedges can be placed underneath the neck to make oral sex easier to perform.

You can get even naughtier by experimenting with bondage furniture: there's everything from beds with specially designed loops to put ties and handcuffs through, to seats with holes cut in them for a woman to sit on while a man performs oral sex. Even if it's a bit out there for you, browsing some of the internet sites offering this furniture will stimulate sexy conversation between you, and could lead to a night of hot fantasy-led sex.

But if all that is a bit extreme, you can go for a more innocent approach. Simply designate one item of furniture in your house as 'the sex place' – it could be a chair or it could be the kitchen table, say. Make love on it sometimes, as an alternative to the bed; neither of you will be able to help grinning when you see a friend innocently sitting in that chair a week later! Having a sexy secret is a good way to bond with your partner: it reinforces the fact that you have something special that only the two of you share.

... *Sofa so good!* ...

Hot Positions

SCORE 5

Kinky Cluedo

Many couples make love in the same place all the time – the bed, all too often.

By taking things outside the bedroom you introduce variety to your sex life,

which helps to keep things fresh. Just make sure that you close the curtains …

TO PLAY

Remember the game Cluedo? This is a naughty version of the same game.

If you have a copy of the game, swap all the room names on the board for actual rooms in your home (and if you don't have the game, stop right here and check out 'Variations of the Game'). 'The Library' can become your kitchen, 'The Ballroom' can become your bedroom, 'The Billiard Room' can become your bathroom, and so on. Next, decide which of your favourite erotic playthings the murder weapons are going to represent. For example, the revolver can represent a set of love balls, the candlestick a candle, the rope a silk scarf and the dagger a vibrator. Only pick toys that you actually have in the house – otherwise, the prize at the end of the game won't be possible.

Now, simply play the game according to the rules, enjoying the anticipation of waiting for your prize. And the prize, of course, is that when the scenario is uncovered you both get to perform the sexy alternative at home using the erotic items represented by the murder weapons.

BENEFITS OF THE GAME

It will get you both chatting openly about different sex acts and the places in which they could theoretically be performed. And who knows – you might get some ideas from the juxtaposition of rooms, props and acts in the game … and, best of all, you get to live them all out.

VARIATIONS OF THE GAME

If you don't have a copy of Cluedo, simply write down – on different pieces of paper – six sexy accessories that you have in the house, six different sex acts and six rooms (if you don't have six rooms, get specific as to which item of furniture in the room is going to be used in the act – for example, the bed or the shower). Pick one of each of the options without looking at them, and hide them.

Divide the remaining slips of paper between the pair of you. Then, work out which act it is, in which room and with which prop. Take it in turns to question each other about the slips of paper you each have – for instance, 'Is it having missionary sex, with a dildo, in the bedroom?' If your partner has any of the acts you've named on their slips of paper, they'll know that you've got at least part of the answer wrong. By questioning each other and listening carefully to each other's answers, you'll be able to work out what the act is through a process of elimination.

... What shall we play? ...

HOT TIP

Most board games can be tailored to have a sexy twist if you have a bit of imagination: with Monopoly, the money earned can be spent of sexual favours rather than just to buy hotels; with Operation, kiss the appropriate part of the body every time you set an alarm off. Dirty-word Scrabble is a fun alternative to the usual kind – just spell out the things that you'd like to happen to you. And as for Buckaroo? Well, you could always try sex 'cowgirl' style with the woman on top!

Build up a collection of sexy items that can be used to add a twist to conventional games: feathers, blindfolds and sex toys are a good start.

Come up with sexy alternatives to the board games in your cupboard, and you'll soon start looking forward to spending rainy Sunday afternoons in together …

Hot Positions

Sitting, standing, lying

Most couples make love in only three different positions: missionary, woman on top and doggie style. This can result in sexual tedium setting in. This game helps you to come up with new positions. Who knows, you could find that they reach parts your usual positions don't …

TO PLAY

Start by rolling a die to select from the following options:

1–2 = sitting

3–4 = standing

5–6 = lying down

Now, depending on what you rolled, pick a sexual position that involves at least one

partner either sitting, standing or lying down. For example, if you roll a 1 or 2, you

could try the sit and spin (man sitting on washing machine, woman sitting on his

lap), seated straddle (man on chair, woman straddling him), or queen for a night

(man in chair, woman sitting astride him with legs thrown over his shoulders).

If you roll a 3 or 4, try The Crane (see page 255), stairway to heaven (woman

standing on step above man, with man standing below, penetrating her) or The

Directory (woman stands on a telephone directory, man penetrates her).

And if you roll a 5 or 6, try classic missionary, the bum lift (missionary with the man raising the woman's buttocks) or on the edge (woman lying with her legs over the edge of the bed, man standing between them).

BENEFITS OF THE GAME

This game encourages you to think outside the norm; after all, most sex tends to happen in bed. By exploring seated and standing positions as well, you're opening up your sex life to more options.

VARIATIONS OF THE GAME

Buy the Kama Sutra or another sex manual and choose six different positions of each type (seated, standing and lying down), then roll a die to pick which one to try.

HOT TIP

Having a hard time coming up with ideas? Here's one of each type of position to choose from:

Standing doggie Ideal for quickies in this position, the woman bends forward from the waist and leans against a wall, while the man penetrates her from behind. Penetration is deep, making it ideal for hitting the G-spot, and the man has plenty of scope to caress the woman's breasts, clitoris and the rest of her body.

Sideways seated The man sits down on a chair and the woman sits side-on, with her legs on the floor or, if it's an armchair, over the side of the chair. She then uses either her hands or her legs to control the thrusting. This stimulates the underside of the penis, in particular the coronal ridge and frenulum, so gives men an extra thrill, and it also offers a different angle of approach. This position is ideal if the man is extremely well endowed, as it controls the level of the penetration.

Right angle The woman lies on her back, keeping one leg straight and raising the other one as high as she can, aiming to rest it on her partner's shoulder. The man kneels between her thighs and penetrates her. The higher the woman's leg, the deeper the penetration, as it lengthens the vagina, making this a great position for G-spot thrills. The man can also easily caress the woman's breasts, torso and clitoris. This position also makes less well-endowed men feel bigger, as it 'tightens' the vagina and gives deep penetration.

... You might want to take this lying down ...

Hot Positions

SCORE 7

Hitting the G

The G-spot is a contentious thing: some scientists claim it's
a myth, but many women are of an opposing view and find that it adds to
their pleasure immensely. This game helps you discover whether or not hitting
the G-spot during sex works for your partner.

TO PLAY

Start by trying to find the G-spot manually (see Hot Tip). Once you've identified it, roll a die to choose from these options:

1 =   doggie

2 =   standing doggie

3 =   bum lift (missionary with the man raising the woman's buttocks)

4 =   on the edge (woman lying with her legs over the edge of the bed, man standing between them)

5 =   wheelbarrow (woman standing on her hands, man standing behind, holding her legs and penetrating her)

6 =   woman on top

Now have sex in the position indicated by the die. All offer deep penetration, making them ideal for G-spot stimulation. While making love, note which position is the most effective, and choose it next time you fancy some G-spot action. (Bear in mind that G-spot stimulation can make some women want to urinate rather than climax, so it may not be for everyone.)

BENEFITS OF THE GAME

G-spot orgasms can be incredibly intense, if a woman is lucky enough to have a sensitive G-spot. Stimulation of the G-spot can also lead to female ejaculation for some women, in which a fluid similar to prostate fluid (of which semen is partly comprised) shoots out. Don't panic if this happens – it has nothing to do with urination and is entirely natural. Some women find that it enhances the experience, some are perturbed by it and others find that it just leaves a bigger wet patch!

VARIATIONS OF THE GAME

Buy a G-spot sex toy and try using it with the woman in different positions to see which makes it easiest to find.

HOT TIP

The G-spot is located on the upper wall of the vagina, and is thought to enhance sexual pleasure for the woman. To find it, slide a finger or two into the vagina and press relatively firmly on the top wall (towards the pubic area rather than towards the bum). There should be a spongy mass about a third of the way up on the upper wall of the vagina that makes the woman tingle when it's touched. If the man doesn't find it at first, he should carry on moving his finger(s) up by about half an inch at a time. Don't worry if it takes a while. The G-spot can be elusive.

If you find the G-spot and want to get really ambitious, you can then move on to finding the A-zone. Discovered in 1996 by scientists investigating vaginal dryness, the Anterior Fornix, or A-zone, is a lesser-known cousin to the G-spot. But, while it may not have received as much attention as the G-spot, once you've found it you'll be amazed you've missed it for so long!

Although the A-zone is best stimulated through sex, get your partner to feel for it with fingers first, to get an idea of where to aim. He should feel for the

G-spot then carry on to the cervix, which feels round. Now, he simply moves the fingers back, halfway between the two points. This is the A-zone.

If it's hit, women will often experience strong contractions, which feel as if they're trying to push their partner out. If this happens, the thing to do is push harder into the woman. It sounds odd, but the harder the thrusting against the A-zone, the better the orgasm will be (although, obviously, if it hurts, don't do it!).

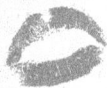

... Ooh – that really hits the spot! ...

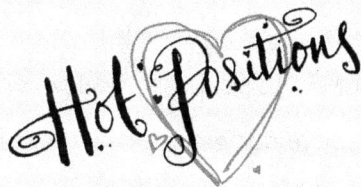

Hot Positions

Size matters

Different positions have different benefits: they can make a man seem larger or smaller, a woman seem tighter or looser. This game shows you how much of an impact a change of position can make – and gives you tricks to incorporate into lovemaking to make it better for both of you.

TO PLAY

Start making love in your favourite sex position. Now, while you're having sex, roll the die and vary what you're doing depending on your roll:

1 = woman brings her legs more tightly together

2 = woman spreads her legs widely

3 = woman raises her left leg

4 = woman raises her right leg

5 = woman flexes her Kegel (vaginal) muscles

6 = woman puts a pillow underneath her hips

Pay attention to the sensation and notice the difference that it makes: does penetration seem deeper or shallower? Does the man's penis seem larger or smaller? Does the woman's vagina seem tighter or is there less friction? By paying attention, you'll know how to vary sex positions in future, should you want more or less sensation of whatever type.

If something doesn't seem to give any benefit, roll the die again and follow the instructions accordingly: different things work for different people, after all.

BENEFITS OF THE GAME

Sometimes, a small tweak is all it takes to turn a good sex position into a great sex position. This game teaches you some of the most common tricks. It also helps you keep things fresh, as you're experimenting with new things together.

VARIATIONS OF THE GAME

Change the die options: for example, the man could lean back on his arms, or hold the woman by the hips. The woman could cross her legs or tighten her buttocks. There are hundreds of tiny ways you can change sex positions, so experiment. You never know what you might discover.

HOT TIP

Certain positions will make a man seem bigger. Two good ones are:

Boosted missionary The woman lies on her back with her legs spread and knees bent. The man lies on top. Once he's slid inside, the woman puts her feet on his thighs or buttocks. He won't have much control over thrusting, as in the traditional missionary position, but penetration is far deeper if the woman bends her legs. The higher up the man's body she puts her feet, the deeper he'll get.

On the edge The woman lies on her back, dangling her legs and thighs over the edge of a bed or other surface, and spreads her legs, resting one on the floor. The man lies on top, with one leg on the floor and the other kneeling on the bed. The woman then wraps the leg that isn't resting on the floor around the man's waist. This deepens penetration.

Other positions will make a man seem smaller. Two good ones are:

Reverse CAT (Coital Alignment Technique) The woman goes on top, taking as much of the man's penis as is comfortable, and gradually moves until she's lying directly on top of him. Both of you gently rock and circle your hips. This stimulates the woman's clitoris and pubic area. If the woman closes her legs it will add intensity for both of you, but the angle means that he won't be able to get every last inch inside.

Flat doggie Rather than kneeling on all fours, the woman lies flat on the bed with the man behind her. He can slide in easily, but penetration is shallower than with traditional doggie, so the woman should find it easier to cope,

... Can you feel the difference?...

Hot Positions

SCORE 9

I have control

Sometimes, the smallest change can make a huge difference to the way that sex feels. In this game, you take it in turns to take control and vary the position you're in to give you the ultimate pleasure. Sometimes it's OK to be selfish.

TO PLAY

Roll a die to decide who's in charge: if it's an odd number, it's the woman, and if it's an even number, it's the man .

Now get into your favourite position, but, rather than starting to have sex, once the man has slid inside the woman, both relax. The partner who's in charge now moves their partner's body into the ideal position: perhaps the man will raise the woman's leg to get deeper penetration, or maybe the woman will push the man's body lower down so that she gets greater clitoral stimulation.

The 'submissive' partner should move as directed by the partner who's in charge. Once the person in charge decides their partner is in the ideal position, start making love.

If you start to fall back into the traditional way you have sex, the 'dominant' partner should move their partner back into the position that gives them the most stimulation.

BENEFITS OF THE GAME

Both of you will get to learn new ways to stimulate your partner during sex. You can use this knowledge to improve sex every time you have it.

VARIATIONS OF THE GAME

Roll a die to pick the starting position, and then follow the rules as above:

1 = missionary   4 = reverse cowgirl

2 = doggie style   5 = spooning

3 = woman on top   6 = standing sex

Play this game regularly, from various starting positions, and with each of you taking turns to be in charge. Before long, you'll have honed all the sex positions in your repertoire to perfection.

HOT TIP

No matter which position you have sex in, some things will make any sexual encounter better.

To start with, have confidence in yourself. There's no point getting het up about your cellulite, belly or other features you're less than proud of. If someone has decided they want to get naked and make love to you, they'll be far too lost in the moment to notice anything other than 'Wow – someone I fancy is naked with me'. Revel in being naked together, and you'll both enjoy it far more.

Don't be scared to ask for what you want, either. If you don't ask, you don't get, but say what you want and your partner will be blown away by your sexual confidence. Even better, they should be more than happy to oblige. If you don't feel comfortable talking dirty, say it with groans. Writhe around when they do things you like, and moan when they hit the spot. Faking orgasm is a bad thing to do, but a bit of exaggeration never went amiss …

Never underestimate grooming, either. Women aren't generally going to be as tempted to get intimate if they know that they'll end up with stubble burn, so shave before you get romantic. And the vast majority of blokes still get all hot under the collar at a glimpse of stocking. Invest in some sexy lingerie – black or red knickers with matching suspenders usually work well, as do seamed stockings or even simple white knickers.

There's no great mystery to sex. If you enjoy it, and aren't ashamed to show that you do, then you'll have a fabulous time together.

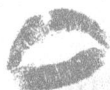

... You're the boss! ...

Hot Positions

Now get creative

Devising your own personalized sexual positions can be

a great way to bond with your partner. How much more intimate is it to have

'our position' than 'our song'? This

game helps you work out a position between you

that hits all of your buttons.

TO PLAY

Roll a die to choose from one of these starting positions:

1 = missionary	4 = reverse cowgirl
2 = doggie style	5 = spooning
3 = woman on top	6 = standing against the wall

Write it down, followed by the words 'then add', and pass the paper to your partner. They write down an addition to the position – for example, if you roll a 1, indicating missionary, your partner could then add 'with left leg raised'. They then add the words 'then add', and pass the paper back to you. You make another addition – for example, 'with hand caressing lower back' – and so on. Take it in turns to make new additions to the position until you both run out of ideas. Then live it out, and see how good the position you've created is.

BENEFITS OF THE GAME

By encouraging you to think about creative additions to your usual lovemaking positions, it will encourage you to be creative when you have sex – whether you're playing the game or not.

You'll also get to learn about the twists you can make to sex that enhance the experience for both of you: for example, if a woman raises her leg, it not only makes penetration deeper but can also make it easier for a man to hit her G-spot.

VARIATIONS OF THE GAME

Rather than starting with a sex position, start with a foreplay act. Make a list of six options – say, cunnilingus, fellatio, hand job, fingering, breast-play or massage. Roll a die to select one, then take it in turns to add a twist to your chosen act.

HOT TIP

Don't just think about ways of moving parts of the body when making your creative additions: it can be fun to incorporate props too. For example, during doggie-style sex, you might find it sexy to include some mild bondage, tying the woman's arms to the head of the bed (NB: only do this with someone you know very well).

During missionary sex, you may find it sexy to drizzle lube over each other's torsos and slide your way to climax together.

In reverse cowgirl (woman on top, facing man's feet), you may choose to add a vibrator to the equation for some double penetration (usual anal-sex rules apply). And, while you're spooning each other, add some decadence by sipping on champagne or feeding each other nibbles as you do so.

Use your imagination, and try to involve all five senses in your lovemaking; it will only intensify the experience.

... Let's twist again ...

Hot Positions

SCORE 11

All change!

Some of the best sexual experiences can come about purely

by chance. In this game, you allow chance to enter into your sex play by

moving from one position to another at the roll

of a die. Just be careful you don't put your back out ...

TO PLAY

Roll a die to choose from one of these starting positions:

1 = missionary   4 = reverse cowgirl

2 = doggie style   5 = spooning

3 = woman on top   6 = standing against the wall

Now, set a timer for 1 minute, get into that position and start having sex. Once the timer goes off, roll the die again to choose from the following options, but don't break contact with each other while you do so:

1 = doggie style   4 = spooning

2 = missionary   5 = reverse cowgirl

3 = standing against the wall   6 = woman on top

The aim of this game is to move from the first position to the second without breaking contact with each other at any point. It may take some time – after all, you don't want to break anything – but you'll be amazed at what's possible if you take things slowly enough.

Once you've successfully moved from the first position to the second position, set the timer for another minute, and have sex until the timer goes off. Then roll a third time to choose from the following options:

1 = standing against the wall   4 = missionary

2 = spooning   5 = woman on top

3 = doggie style   6 = reverse cowgirl

Move into that position – again, without breaking contact. Once you get into the third position, you can then have sex as normal (no more timer!). But make sure you remember all the interesting positions you encountered while you were getting there …

BENEFITS OF THE GAME

A lot of the time, great sex happens on the spur of the moment, and you can discover new thrills purely by rolling around and having fun. This game uses the random nature of rolling a die to simulate that fun romping around.

VARIATIONS OF THE GAME

Buy a sex manual or ancient text like the Kama Sutra and make your own lists of sex positions to choose from. Set the timer for 5 minutes rather than 1 minute if the man goes for hours, and set it for only 30 seconds if he reaches climax somewhat quicker.

You can also stop midway through trying to get into your second (or third) position if you find one that really hits the spot for both of you. After all, that is one of the things that great sex is all about.

HOT TIP

Having a laugh in the bedroom is a good way to keep your love life fresh, and romping around from one position to another, as this game allows, will help you both keep that sense of fun going.

Tickle fights are another entertaining way to end up in all sorts of compromising positions. Use your fingers or even a feather; the loser, of course, has to pay a sexual forfeit. If one of you is more ticklish than the other, it just means you have to search all the harder.

Or, try blowing raspberries on each other's stomach, dirty dancing in the bedroom together, or even dressing up in each other's undies to add a sense of fun to what you're doing. You may feel silly, but couples who can laugh together tend to have much more successful relationships – and you never know, you could discover a new kinky thrill at the same time, too.

... Let's have a laugh ...

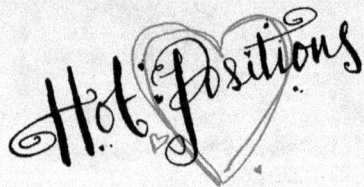

Hot Positions

Dirty Pictionary

Talking about your favourite positions will help you learn

more about what turns your partner on, but it can be hard

to do. This game introduces a fun element to make the conversation easier.

Just make sure that you use what

you've learned after the game ends.

TO PLAY

For this game, you'll need two pads of paper, a pen and a timer. Start by rolling a die to determine who goes first: if it's an odd number, the man goes first, and if it's an even number, the woman goes first.

The person who is going first writes down their favourite sex position on a piece of paper, out of view from their partner, folds it in half and puts it to one side. This stage is to prevent cheating. They then turn over the timer and start drawing their favourite sex position. Their partner has to guess what the position is before a minute is up. If they guess correctly, they score a point, to be redeemed against sexual favours later.

Once the time has run out, the other person then takes their turn, and draws their favourite sex position for their partner to guess. Continue to take it in turns until you've both written your top five positions, and have a choice of ten sexual positions to decide between for the night. The person with the highest score gets to choose the position, of course.

BENEFITS OF THE GAME

You get to learn about each other's favourite sex positions in a fun and non-threatening way.

VARIATIONS OF THE GAME

Rather than drawing a sexual position, draw another type of sex act instead: oral sex, manual sex or even some kind of fantasy or fetish instead. Bear in mind, though, that it could take all your artistic skills if you've got an elaborate 'landlord and wanton wench'-style fantasy!

HOT TIP

It's common for couples to have different favourite sexual positions. If this is the case with you – say, the man loves woman on top, while the woman prefers doggie-style sex – the only answer is compromise. Don't let the dominant partner always insist on their favourite position, as this can lead to both of you having reduced libidos (for one of you because you're having sex in a position that doesn't really do it for you, and for the other because your partner is never that enthusiastic about sex).

See if there's a position that, while not being number one for either of you, is something that you both enjoy. Or take it in turns to have sex in each other's favourite position, and think if there are any ways that you can enhance it for yourself. For example, masturbating during sex can make it easier for a woman to come. By working together, you'll have the best sex.

... I'll tell you mine if you tell me yours ...

Hot Positions

Vice versa

It's easy to settle into your own favourite position during sex: always lying back and letting your partner do the work, or preferring to go on top every time. By breaking your usual habits, you can inject fresh passion into your sex life, which can only be a good thing.

TO PLAY

Start by writing down the position that you most like being in when you're hav-ing sex – for example, lying on your back, kneeling or lying on your side. Your partner should do the same thing.

Next, both of you should swap pieces of paper and assume whichever posi-tion your partner has written down. Now comes the potentially tricky bit. Between you, figure out a sex position that accommodates both of the posi-tions you wrote down.

For example, if both of you wrote 'lying on my back', the woman could lie flat on her back on top of her partner, while he thrusts inside her. If the woman wrote 'kneeling' and the man wrote 'lying on my back', then the man could kneel while the woman lies flat on her back on the bed, with the man raising her hips to penetrate her. And if the woman wrote 'sitting up' and the man wrote 'kneeling', the man can sit with the woman straddling him while she kneels (don't forget that you're swapping pieces of paper and assuming your partner's position).

BENEFITS OF THE GAME

By each of you assuming the other's favourite position, you will get out of any ruts that you may have got into. This game also encourages you to think more creatively about the sex positions that you adopt.

VARIATIONS OF THE GAME

Don't swap pieces of paper. Instead, both get into your favourite position, and then figure out a way to incorporate these into a sex position that suits you both.

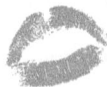

... So how do you want me? ...

HOT TIP

Some positions can be pretty difficult to achieve if you and your partner are of radically different sizes and/or heights. However, with a little bit of imagination you should still be able to add variety to your sex life.

If one partner is significantly taller than the other, but you want to have sex standing up, judicious use of stairs or a telephone directory (or two) can help. You could even stand on a sofa if there's a huge difference in size!

If a man is particularly plump, try positions in which the woman is bending over in front of him, as this will help him lift his stomach out of the way. And if the woman's particularly plump, try sex with the woman lying with her hips dangling over the edge of the bed and the man standing between her legs, thrusting.

If either of you has a bad back, be careful about any position that puts too much strain on it – like sex standing up, for instance. Using furniture to help make things easier.

Hot Positions

Spice it up

Making minor changes to your usual positions can spice

things up, but it can be hard to think of exactly how. In this game, you let the

die decide exactly how you're going

to move. Give your sex life over to chance …

TO PLAY

First, roll a die to establish your starting position:

      1 = standing against the wall   4 = missionary

      2 = spooning   5 = woman on top

      3 = doggie style   6 = reverse cowgirl

Roll again – this time to see what the objective of the sex session is (other than the obvious!):

      1 = clitoral stimulation   4 = kissing while having sex

      2 = breast stimulation   5 = caressing the man's

                                      testicles during sex

      3 = deep penetration   6 = caressing the woman's

                                      back during sex

Between you, figure out a way to have sex in the selected position while achieving the objective given. For example, if you roll a 2, for spooning, followed by a 5, for caressing the man's testicles, the woman could reach between her own legs while the man penetrates her, to achieve this goal. If you roll a 3 for dog-gie-style sex and then a 2 for breast stimulation, the man can cup the woman's breasts while they have sex. Or if you roll a 4 for missionary, followed by a 3 for deep penetration, the woman can put a pillow under her hips or the man can pull her hips upwards with his hands during sex.

BENEFITS OF THE GAME

This game helps you think about the benefits of each different sex position, which in turn will help you stimulate each other in the best ways during your usual sex sessions.

VARIATIONS OF THE GAME

Make your own lists of options tailored to your own desires: for example, you may wish to add anal stimulation or even spanking to your options.

HOT TIP

Clitoral stimulation is generally the key to female orgasm, and the design of the male and female body doesn't always make it easy for the relevant bits to touch. However, trying Coital Alignment Technique, or CAT, is sure to get you purring.

CAT is a variation on the most popular sexual position: the missionary. The woman lies on her back with legs slightly apart and bent. The man lies on top but, instead of resting his weight on his elbows, he rests his full weight on the woman. If he's particularly heavy, he should lean slightly to one side and hold some of his weight on one arm.

Next, the man shuffles forward so that his pelvis is directly on top of his partner's. She then wraps her legs around him, keeping them relatively straight, so that her ankles are more or less around his calves. Now, both partners start grinding. The woman should press up as the man moves backwards, so that both of you are rocking gently against one another, and stimulating each other softly but also directly.

As orgasm approaches, rather than speeding up, just keep gently rocking so that the orgasm comes naturally rather than being 'chased'.

As well as offering fantastic clitoral stimulation, this position is great if a man suffers from premature ejaculation, as the sensation is less intense for him. You can always change to a different position – doggie style is number one for a lot of men – so that he can have his orgasm afterwards.

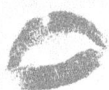

... Ooh – that's purrfect ...

Hot Positions

SCORE 15

Freeze-frame

Sexy films can be a great way to enhance your sex life, if you're both

comfortable watching them. This game takes the film and makes it interactive.

It will decide how you're going

to make love tonight. And, after watching it together, you

may even be aroused enough to skip foreplay!

TO PLAY

To play this game, you'll need a sexy film on video or DVD. If you don't like the idea of traditional adult films, try something specifically designed for couples, like the Lovers' Guide series.

Now, each write a number between 0 and 60 on a bit of paper. Put the counter display on on your video/DVD player, and fast-forward until you reach the first of the two numbers – so, if your partner wrote down 10 and you wrote down 15, fast-forward to 10 minutes in. Now, write down the position that the man and the woman are both in; if they aren't involved in something sexual, fast-forward until the first point afterwards that they are.

Next, fast-forward to your partner's number – in this case, 15 minutes. Again, write down the position that both the man and the woman are in.

This is where things start getting really interesting. The man assumes the position that the man was in on-screen when you first stopped the film. The woman assumes the position that the woman was in on-screen when you stopped the film for the second time. You now both have to figure out together how you can have sex without moving from the positions that each of you are in.

BENEFITS OF THE GAME

Many couples find that sexy films are a good way to fire up wilting libidos. They can provide erotic ideas as well as act as foreplay. Don't just think of them as a male thing, either: research has shown that women get just as physically aroused as men do by erotic films.

VARIATIONS OF THE GAME

If you don't have a video or DVD player (or any erotic films), use a sex manual instead. Flick to a page and act out whatever is recommended on that page.

HOT TIP

Adult films used to be targeted primarily at men, but these days there are more and more series aimed at women and couples. From educational videos/DVDs to more hardcore action (but produced by a woman), you should be able to find something that turns you both on.

One of the easiest ways to find out what does it for both of you – without spending a fortune – is to spend some time surfing adult sites on the internet together. That way, you can see the type of action that appeals – and, conversely, discover any top turn-offs. For example, one of you may not want to watch anal sex while the other may find it a huge turn on. Unless both of you find a film arousing, don't watch it together!

Once you've found something that turns you both on, you can continue the experience online, either by downloading films from specially designed internet sites or by visiting one of many online sex shops designed for women and cou-ples. Even amazon.co.uk has a selection of erotic videos and DVDs nowadays, so don't get in a panic that you'll have to go to any sleazy websites.

So, now that you've got a film you both enjoy, and it's been delivered to your door, it's time to make a sexy evening of it. Have a sensual bath together, and maybe even make some aphrodisiac snacks to feed each other with teasingly while you watch the film together. Make sure that condoms, lube, sex toys and anything else that you might want to use during lovemaking are within easy reach of the sofa: that way, you can emulate the action on-screen while indulging in your own X-rated action.

... Let's fast-forward to the good bits! ...

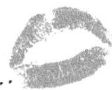

Hot Positions

Torrid Twister

Of all the children's board games, Twister is probably the most commonly abused for sexual purposes. And rightly so! A game of naked Twister will help you get into all manner of positions you've never dreamed of before – or, if you have, only in your raunchiest dreams …

TO PLAY

In order to play this game, you ideally need a copy of the board game Twister. If you have one, the rules are incredibly simple (otherwise, see below). Get undressed and then simply play the game as instructed. Spin the spinner and put whatever body part it directs onto the correctly coloured dot. You'll end up in all manner of lewd positions – and what you do when you're in them is entirely up to you.

If you don't own a copy of Twister, you can still play this game – it just takes a little more preparation. Simply get a very large piece of paper – wallpaper will do – and use felt- tips to draw even numbers of red, yellow, green, purple, black and blue circles on it, evenly spaced. Now, roll a die to determine which colour you have to aim for:

1 = red	3 = green	5 = black
2 = yellow	4 = purple	6 = blue

Roll the die again to establish which body part you have to put on the spot:

1 = right foot	3 = right hand	5 = right elbow
2 = left foot	4 = left hand	6 = left elbow

Take it in turns to roll the die, and see how entangled you end up getting.

BENEFITS OF THE GAME

You'll laugh together, and end up in positions you'd never have imagined.

VARIATIONS OF THE GAME

Write lists of ruder body parts – left nipple, right buttock or left testicle, for example – then play the game as above.

HOT TIP

If you enjoy playing adult Twister, take a lead from the so-called 'Mazola parties' that were rumoured to happen in 1960s America. Participants would strip off, spread a large plastic sheet on the ground and then tackle each other. To further lubricate proceedings, each contender was coated in oil.

Obviously, getting the neighbours involved isn't what the suggestion is! But adding oil to a game of naked Twister can make things even steamier. So, before you start playing Twister, give each other an erotic – and very oily – massage. Using aphrodisiac aromatherapy oils like sandalwood or ylang ylang will add an extra level of eroticism to proceedings. Then, when you're both suitably covered in oil, start playing.

The advantage of using oil is that it helps you slide sensually against one another, in a way that feels totally different from normal skin-to-skin contact.

If you don't have any massage oil to hand, soap suds can also provide a sexy sliding sensation: start by showering together and soaping each other all over, but don't wash the soap suds off before you start playing the game. Make sure that you lay down towels wherever you're going to be playing, so that you don't soak the furniture, and turn the heating on so that you don't end up shivering in the wrong way. Also, be careful that the soap suds don't get into your more intimate areas, as they could cause irritation.

If you're planning on having penetrative sex – which, let's face it, after sliding against each other for an entire game of Twister, is probably highly likely – use lube instead of oil or soap, as a condom-safe alternative.

... 'You put your left foot in ...'

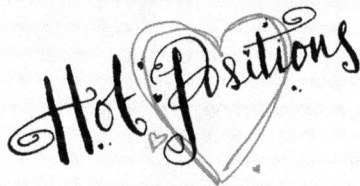

Hot Positions

SCORE 17

Master and slave

Often, in couples, one partner will be more sexually confident, usually initiating the action, while the other partner is more passive. In this game, you take it in turns to swap roles and dictate who does what, and to whom. How better to find out what your partner really wants?

TO PLAY

Start by rolling a die to determine who gets to be the 'master' and who gets to be the 'slave'. If you roll an odd number, the woman gets to be master, and if you roll an even number, the man gets to be master.

Once you've determined who's who, the master orders the slave to have sex in a position of their choosing, and the slave follows orders …

BENEFITS OF THE GAME

Most couples tend to fall into their own roles, with one person as dominant and the other submissive, even if this only entails one partner always initiating sex. By exchanging roles, you will widen your sexual scope, and could discover a hidden sexual side to yourself.

VARIATIONS OF THE GAME

Expand the master-and-slave relationship to cover a wider variety of sexual acts. For example, the master may demand the slave gives a massage lasting at least 20 minutes, or could get kinkier and administer a spanking to the slave – as long as it's something that both of you are happy to try. The slave must follow any orders given. However, bear in mind that this is about role-play, not forcing your partner to do something against their will, so don't pick anything that you know your partner will hate.

If you want to go really wild, you could incorporate appropriate clothing – leatherwear or tight black clothes, for example – to the game. Or you may even want to add some props, such as nipple clamps. Make sure that you're both very aware of each other's limits, though – and if in doubt, don't.

HOT TIP

The master-and-slave game can be considered to be a form of sub/dom and, as such, you should make sure that you have a 'safe' word in place. This is a word that allows the submissive partner to stop any situation or action at any time. Saying 'no' and 'stop' can be considered to be part of the fun of sex games involving control, so they are best avoided. Instead, some people use the colour terms yellow (slow down, ease off – that's too much!) and red (stop now!), while others use something completely random of their own choosing. Whatever safe word you choose, use it consistently, and as soon as you feel remotely uncomfortable.

If you choose to incorporate any form of spanking or more intense pain into proceedings, it's important to help your partner 'come down' afterwards: the master should cuddle the slave and reassure them that they are loved, and possibly even run them a bath or give them a massage. Not only will this help you both get back into your 'normal' roles, but it will also help counter the chemicals that will be running naturally through your partner's body: pain-play and humiliation both create an endorphin rush, which can feel great at the time, but has a subsequent come-down.

The golden rule with any kind of power-play is that it should stop the second that either partner feels uncomfortable: it's not always the slave who feels bad – some people find it traumatic to be dominant. It should only be something explored by couples who are secure in their relationship and know each other well, and is not something to try in a casual relationship, as it requires trust.

... What does Master bid me do? ...

Hot Positions

Tied-up tease

It's amazing how creative people can get when there are obstacles to be

overcome. This game uses this human trait

to your advantage. By introducing a degree of restriction, you'll need to use

your imagination to devise a solution –

and a new position at the same time.

TO PLAY

First, roll a die to decide which partner gets tied up: if it's an odd number, it's the man, and if it's an even number, then it's the woman.

Now, roll another die to choose from the following list of body parts:

1 = left arm	3 = ankles	5 = wrists
2 = right arm	4 = elbows	6 = thumbs

This is the body part that will be tied – only you get to decide how to tie it (whether to the head of the bed, or to another body part, say). For example, if you roll a 3 then a 1, the man could have his left arm tied to his leg, or could have it tied above his head to the bed. Whatever you choose, do make sure that you don't tie it too tightly, as this can cut off the blood flow and be dangerous. And **never** tie anything around the neck, as this can be fatal.

Once you have tied your partner, they need to think of a way in which you can have sex. The tied person should be the one who takes the lead, as they know what will be comfortable. Then, you simply have sex as directed by the tied partner.

BENEFITS OF THE GAME

This game helps you get creative about the sex positions you use: if someone's elbow is tied to their thigh, it's difficult to just have sex missionary style!

VARIATIONS OF THE GAME

Leave the decision entirely to the die: roll twice, with the first die-roll selecting the first body part, and the second deciding what that body part will be tied to. Use your common sense, though, and don't tie your partner up in such a way as to make them uncomfortable. Once tied, check that your partner's breathing is OK, and untie them straight away if they get pins and needles. Always make sure that you can release someone quickly when they're tied: keep scissors within reach, and untie them the second they ask.

... This one's bound to be fun ...

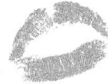

HOT TIP

No matter what position you're in, toned Kegels (vaginal muscles) will enhance the experience for both of you. Kegel exercises were designed to help women tone up their pelvic floor muscles; practised regularly, they make it easier for a woman to reach orgasm, and also increase the intensity.

One of the easiest ways for a woman to find her pelvic floor muscles is for her to sit on the toilet, start to urinate, then stop the flow of urine, and repeat this until she gets used to contracting the right group of muscles. Another way is to insert a finger into the vagina, then tighten the muscles around it.

When doing Kegel exercises, slowly contract the muscles, hold for a count of three and relax for a count of three. Try five repetitions each day to begin with, and gradually work up to as many as can be done without discomfort.

Once a woman is adept at squeezing, she can move to 'pulsing'. Ten rapid squeezes lasting only a second or so will feel good too, and can even result in an orgasm!

Once a woman's Kegels are toned, there are numerous ways to enhance sex. The man can enter fully, then stay still as the woman pulses her muscles to 'milk' an orgasm out of him.

Alternatively, the man can enter the woman, but only by about a centimetre. She can then use her muscles to pull him inside slowly. All she needs to do is clench, then release, and repeat until his full length is inside. Be warned: this can 'suck' condoms off, so don't try this unless you've both been tested and can safely practise sex without a condom.

ONE LAST TRICK: HOW TO ALWAYS WIN!

If you want to make sure that you always win at a game, there's a cheat that you can use to get your own way. Only use it in jest, though – otherwise you're not being fair on your partner.

One little-known fact is that the opposite sides of a die always total 7. If you throw a pair, then, the total of both top numbers added to both bottom numbers will always be 14. Use this to your advantage.

Start by writing down the number 14 on a piece of paper (or somewhere on your body) without your partner seeing. Now, ask them to roll the dice and add both bottom numbers to both top numbers. Bet them that you know what 'random' number they will produce before they even roll the dice – and, of course, if you're right, they have to perform a forfeit …

This principle can also be used to particularly impressive effect by teaming it with a watch. Ask your partner to look at a clock or watch and secretly pick any of the numbers 1 to 12. Tell them to then look at the number directly opposite that one (so if they picked 9 that would be 3, 11 would be 5, and so on) and subtract the smaller number from the larger. Whatever number they end up with, tell them to add 1 to that to give them their special magic number. Bet them that you can reveal their magic number with a single roll of the die; if you're right, they have to perform a lascivious act on you. Now, roll the die, add the top and bottom numbers, and – hey presto! – it reveals their magic number as … 7. And you get to win the game – and your ultimate desire.

And finally

Now that you've reached the end of the book, you should have learned a lot about your partner: their favourite foreplay techniques, sexual positions and fantasies. And they should have learned a lot about how best to please you, whether in the way they talk to you, the way that they touch you, or a combination of both.

But don't let it stop there. Continue talking with your partner about sex: people's tastes change as time goes on, and what suits somebody a year into a relationship may have lost its appeal five years down the line.

You shouldn't have to rely on playing games to find out what your partner wants; they're just a useful way to help open up communication channels between the pair of you. And if you keep talking openly about what you like in bed, you'll be more likely to get it!

Don't rely solely on this book for sexy games, either: different couples enjoy different things, so devise some games that appeal to your own particular quirks. Perhaps you'll want to play games involving lingerie, public sex (careful, as generally speaking it's illegal) or spanking. Maybe you'd prefer something that focuses on more romantic elements – cuddling, moonlit walks or making love on a beach. So, start writing those lists and rolling the die to choose what to go for. Adapt the games in this book to incorporate your own favourite activities, or look at the board games you have in your house and see if you can add a sexy twist by using your imagination.

Remember: couples who play and laugh together are building bonds, communicating and having fun. You can explore each other's minds and bodies through these games – and no doubt have some fantastic orgasms while you're doing so. What more could you want to boost your relationship?

One thing is for sure: if you've worked your way through every game in this book, you are now a better lover than when you first started – and you will have developed your relationship with your partner, too. Who says playing games is frivolous?

FURTHER READING

The Dating Survival Guide: The Top Ten Tactics for Total Success,
   Dr Pam Spurr, Robson Books, UK, 2002
Sex Tips for Girls, Flic Everett, Channel 4 books, UK, 2002
The Big Bang, Emma Taylor and Lorelei Sharkey, Hodder, 2004
Tickle Your Fancy: A Woman's Guide to Sexual Self-Pleasure, Sadie Allison,
   Tickle Kitty Press, US, 2001
My Secret Garden: Women's Sexual Fantasies, Nancy Friday, Quartet
   Books Ltd, US, 2001
My Secret Garden Shed: True-life Male Sexual Fantasies, edited by
   Paul Scott, Nexus, UK, 2002
Why Men Lie and Women Cry, Allan and Barbara Pease, Orion Books,
   UK, 2002

Also by the author

The Lovers' Guide Lovemaking Deck, Connections, UK, 2004
Brief Encounters: The Essential Guide to Casual Sex, Fusion, UK, 2005
Things a Woman Should Know About Seduction, Prion, UK, 2005

RESOURCES

Websites

www.cliterati.co.uk Erotic story website designed for women

www.LoversGuide.com Love and sex advice, video clips and more

www.ScarletMagazine.co.uk Sex magazine for women, with sensual stories
and honest, feisty advice

www.LoveHoney.co.uk Sex toys, lingerie and everything else you might want
to spice up your evening

www.theeroticbookshop.co.uk Every erotic book and sex manual you can
imagine is here

http://www.scarleteen.com Designed for teenagers but suitable for adults
too: honest, interesting and detailed information about every aspect of sex
and relationships

www.sauce-goddess.co.uk Erotic photography service for women and
couples, run by a woman and based in London

Videos/DVDs

The Lovers' Guide: Sex Positions Over 50 different positions explained

The Lovers' Guide: Sexplay Everything you ever wanted to know about foreplay

The Lovers' Guide: Seven Keys to Sensational Sex How to keep the sparkle
there from first date to forever

ACKNOWLEDGEMENTS

Thanks to: my family, for being understanding, as always, about me writing about sex for a living; Sarah Hedley, my editorial partner-in-crime at Scarlet magazine and the only person I know who's tested as many sex toys as I have, for helping me devise games when my brain was failing, calming me down when my stress levels reached fever-pitch, and generally being a great mate; Mil Millington, for storing back-ups of all my files and making sure I didn't lose the book midway through writing it; and for reading through to make sure I hadn't suggested anything too ridiculous; Paul Zenon, for giving me the dice tricks in the conclusion. And, of course, my fab agent Chelsey Fox, and everyone at Eddison Sadd, in particular Ian Jackson, for being a joy to deal with.

EDDISON•SADD EDITIONS

Editorial Director Ian Jackson
Proofreader Nikky Twyman
Art Director Elaine Partington
Mac Designer Malcolm Smythe
Production Sarah Rooney and Nick Eddison

www.ingramcontent.com/pod-product-compliance
Lightning Source LLC
Chambersburg PA
CBHW051951270326
41929CB00015B/2611